AF663935

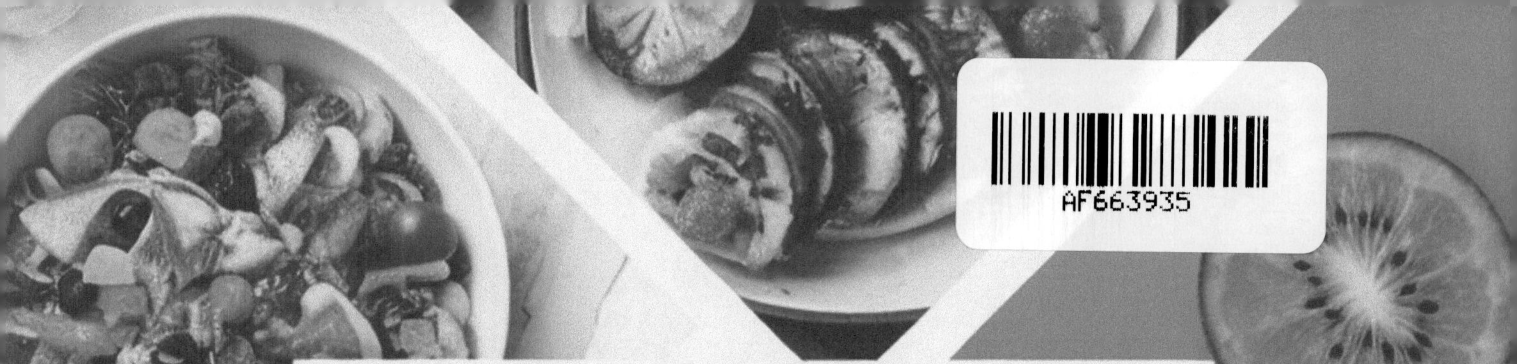

THE EASY AND TASTY

DASH DIET

COOKBOOK

FOR SENIORS

THE COMPLETE 30-DAY MEAL PLAN TO LOWER BLOOD PRESSURE NATURALLY WITH DELICIOUS, QUICK, AND EASY LOW-SODIUM RECIPES.

ELIZA THORNWELL

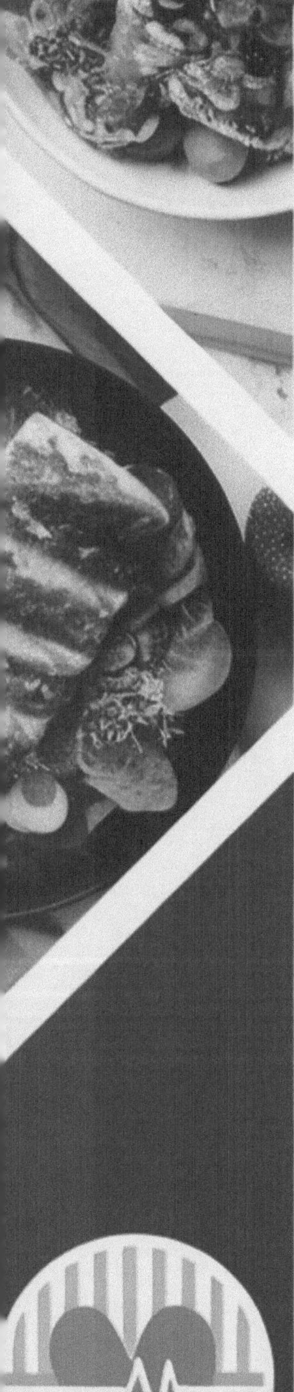

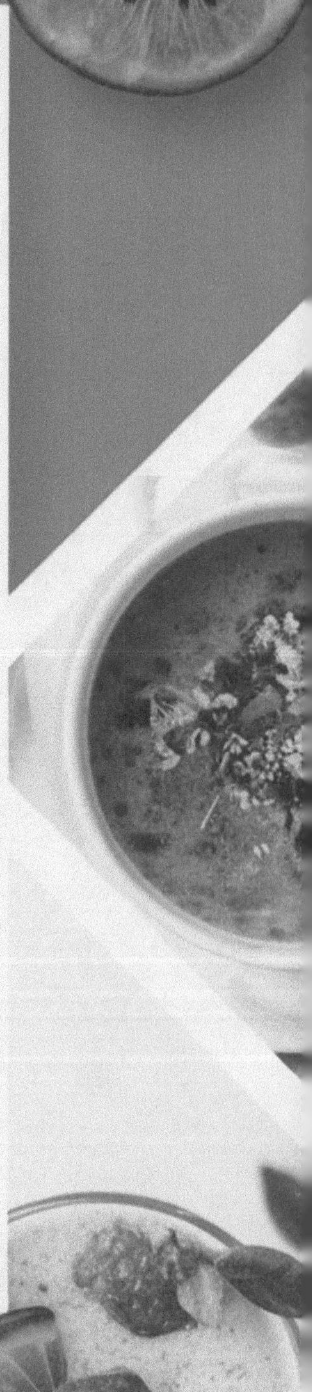

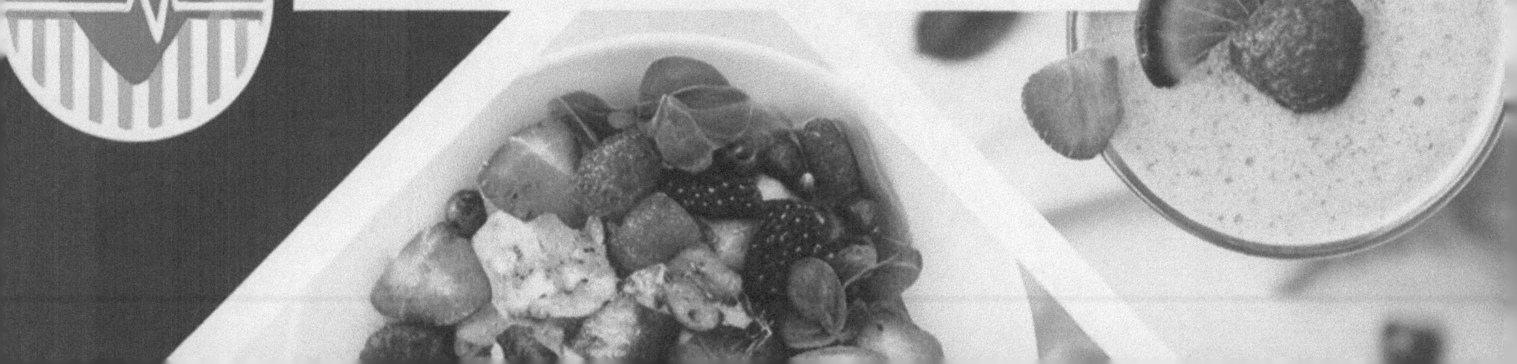

Published by

GRAPEVINE BOOKS

www.grapevinebooks.com

email: contact@grapevinebooks.com

Ordering Information:

Quantity sales: Special discounts are

available on quantity purchases

by corporations, associations, and others.

For details, reach out to the publisher.

First published by Grapevine Books, 2025

Copyright © Grapevine, 2025

All rights reserved

CONTENTS

THE DASH DIET

BREAKFAST

1. Vegetable and Feta Cheese Scramble
2. Zucchini Mix Muffins
3. Easy Chive Omelet
4. Oatmeal Rest
5. Fruit Green Smoothie
6. Banana and Oats Muffins
7. Spicy Tomato and Herb Baked Eggs
8. Strawberry and Yogurt Parfait
9. Breakfast Barley with Banana & Honey
10. Broccoli and Parsley Omelet
11. Cinnamon Flavored Apple Granola
12. Spinach and Eggs Florentine
13. Twin Berry Parfait
14. Early Morning Fruit Crunch
15. Easy Egg Sandwich
16. Honey Mixed Oats Granola
17. Broccoli, Onion and Carrot Omelet
18. Pumpkin Mix Pancakes
19. Cheese Mini Egg and Broccoli Omelet
20. Blueberry Double Pancakes

APPETIZERS & SNACKS

1. Fiesta Surprise Roll
2. Bean Dip and Olive Athenos
3. Stuffed Quesadillas
4. Sesame Hummus
5. Roasted Almonds with Rosemary
6. White Bean and Nut Dip
7. Peach and Raspberry Lassi
8. Wafers and Cinnamon Snack Mix
9. Pumpkin Vanilla Smoothie
10. Snack Curry Mix
11. Popcorn Snack Mix
12. Apple Buttermilk and Oat Bran Muffins
13. Sweet Wheat Muffins
14. Zucchini Cinnamon Muffins
15. Roasted Chickpea Pancakes
16. Golden Potato Pancakes

LUNCH

1. Swiss Apple Panini
2. Vegetarian Pasta Soup
3. Grilled Veggie Toast Californian-Style
4. Tuna Salad Tuscan-Style
5. Delightful Tortellini Salad
6. Healthy Tuna Salad
7. Avocado, Strawberry & Melon Salad
8. Cheesy Pear & Turkey Sandwich
9. Chunky Tomato Spaghetti Squash
10. Pita Pizza
11. Mushroom, Tofu & Spinach Soba Mix
12. Salmon Salad in a Pita
13. Skillet Potatoes and Sausage
14. Rice Bowl, Southwest-Style
15. Sirloin Potage
16. Shrimp, Corn & Raspberry Salad
17. Black Bean & Guacamole Cake
18. Shrimp, Cherry Tomato & Asparagus Salad
19. Cheesy Mushroom & Spinach Wraps
20. Taco Chicken Salad
21. Sunshine in a Wrap
22. Delicious Millet Cakes
23. Quesadillas & Cilantro-Yogurt Dip
24. Roast Chicken Dahl Curry

DINNER

1. Lemon Garlic Baked Salmon
2. Mediterranean Chickpea Stew
3. Garlic Herb Chicken with Spinach
4. Sweet Potato and Lentil Curry
5. Baked Cod with Tomatoes
6. Turkey and Veggie Stir-Fry
7. Herb and Lemon Chicken Quinoa Bowl
8. Creamy Spinach Stuffed Peppers
9. Salmon and Asparagus Foil Pack
10. Chicken and Vegetable Soup
11. Mushroom Barley Risotto
12. Balsamic Glazed Chicken
13. Lentil and Spinach Soup

14. Turkey Meatballs with Tomato Basil Sauce
15. Baked Tilapia with Herbs
16. Vegetable Brown Rice Pilaf
17. Shrimp and Spinach Stir-Fry
18. Stuffed Eggplant with Quinoa
19. Lemon Herb Chicken and Broccoli
20. Tofu and Vegetable Skillet
21. Garlic Shrimp with Zucchini Noodles
22. Hearty Chicken and Sweet Corn Stew
23. Baked Stuffed Tomatoes
24. Lemon Herb Tilapia with Green Beans
25. Veggie and Brown Rice Casserole
26. Turkey and Spinach Skillet
27. Honey Dijon Chicken with Broccoli
28. Vegetable Lentil Shepherd's Pie
29. Broiled Citrus Herb Salmon
30. Mediterranean Chicken with Couscous

SLOW COOKER

1. Lemon Crock Pot Chicken
2. Turkey Chili
3. Crock Pot Chicken, Rice & Veggie Soup
4. Crock Pot Honey Pecan Chicken
5. Sweet & Sour Crock Pot Chicken Over Brown Rice
6. Crock Pot Apple Cinnamon Oatmeal
7. Mushroom Barley Crock Pot Risotto
8. Crock Pot Chicken Cacciatore
9. Crock Pot Pea & Ham Soup
10. Crock Pot Barbeque Chicken
11. Crock Pot Pork Chops with Creamy Sauce
12. Crock Pot Chicken Tortilla Soup
13. Crock Pot Venison & Vegetables
14. Roast Crock Pot Chicken
15. Crock Pot Ground Chicken & Brown Rice
16. Crock Pot Pacific Chicken
17. Crock Pot Seafood Stew
18. Barbeque Pulled Pork Roast
19. Crock Pot Mac 'N Cheese (Light)
20. Irish Bean & Cabbage Crock Pot Stew

DESSERTS

1. Cinnamon & Almond Rice Pudding
2. Stuffed & Baked Apples
3. Watermelon & Lemon Sorbet
4. Blueberry & Blackberry Yogurt Popsicles
5. Pumpkin Whip
6. Baked Blueberry Bling
7. Pina Colada Popsicles
8. Berry-Banana Guilt-Free Ice Cream
9. Melon & Orange Slushy
10. Summer Berries in Frozen Yogurt
11. Cranberry-Watermelon Agua Fresca
12. Fresh Strawberries & Honey Yogurt
13. Almond & Tahini Cookies
14. Sweet Potato Pie
15. Apple Crumble Pie
16. Orange Rice Pudding

DRINKS

1. Berry Mix Smoothie
2. Soy Fruit Smoothie
3. Cantaloupe and Orange Smoothie
4. Green Tea and Cranberry Smoothie
5. Orange Strawberry Twirl
6. Berry Orange Mix
7. Smoothie Sunray
8. Date and Almond Shake
9. Mango and Avocado Smoothie Surprise
10. Not Too Sweet Blueberry Smoothie
11. Golden Iced Latte
12. Minty Iced Tea
13. Breakfast Mojito
14. Spicy Tomato Sipper

DAILY MEAL PLANNER

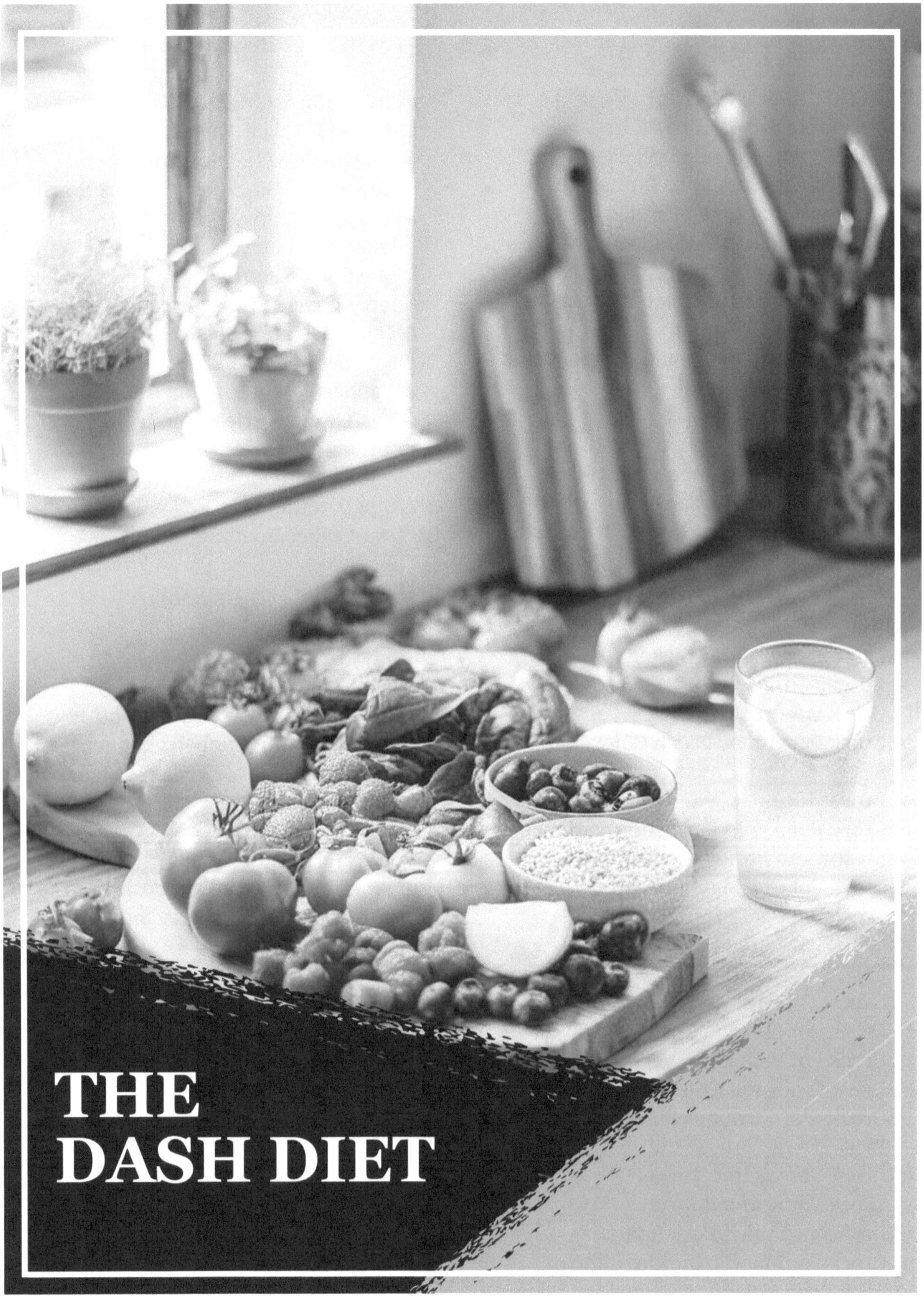

THE DASH DIET

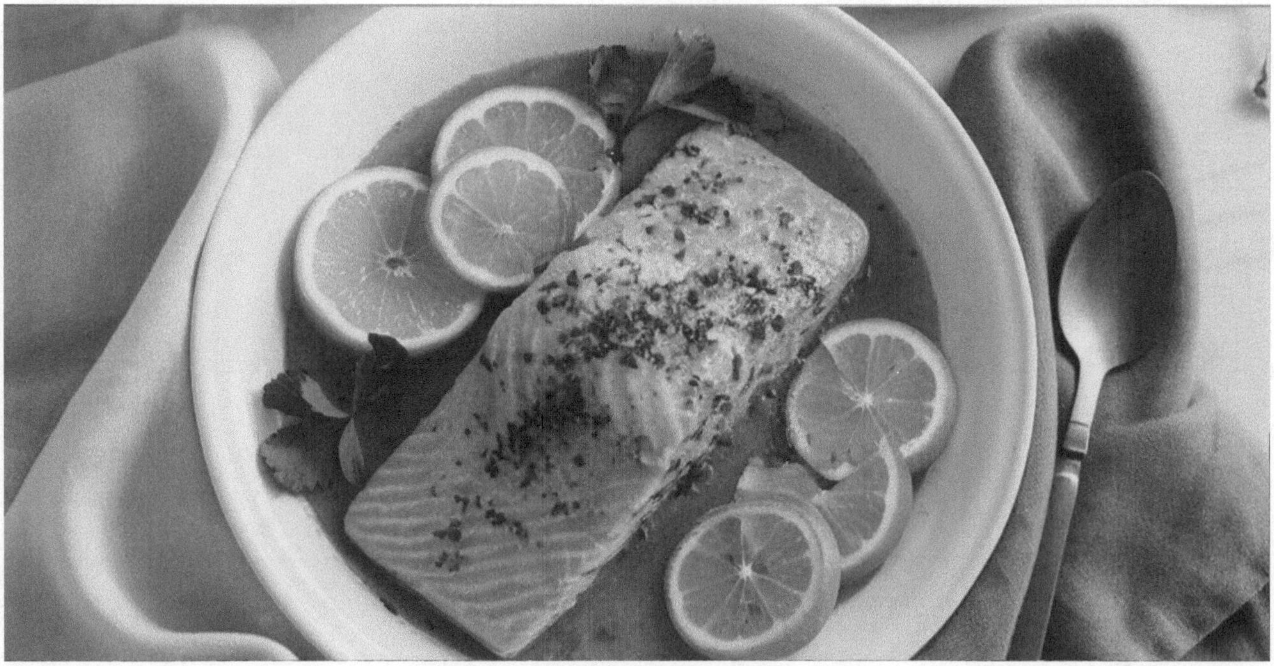

A NEW BEGINNING

At 72, Margaret felt like she had tried everything. Her blood pressure pills had multiplied over the years, and she was constantly being told to cut back—on salt, bread, even fruit. She missed the joy of eating. Every doctor's visit ended the same way: another warning, another pill, and another frustrated sigh.

Then one day, her daughter handed her a copy of this very DASH Cookbook. It wasn't another strict diet or confusing plan. This guide finally made sense. Within a few weeks, Margaret noticed her blood pressure dropping, her energy returning, and her meals becoming something to look forward to again. That transformation is exactly what I want for you.

What if taking care of your health didn't mean giving up the joy of eating well? What if, instead of counting calories or cutting out everything you love, you could lower your blood pressure while enjoying every bite?

Many readers come to me feeling tired, confused, and overwhelmed by all the conflicting advice out there. You might be one of them, searching for a way to take care of your heart without giving up the joy of food or the comfort of a warm, satisfying dinner.

This book was created for people like you, real people who want to live better, feel better, and eat better. And that's exactly what the DASH diet delivers.

It's not a list of restrictions or rigid rules. It's a flexible, realistic, and science-backed plan built to fit your life. My goal isn't just to help you eat better. My goal is to help you feel better, every single day.

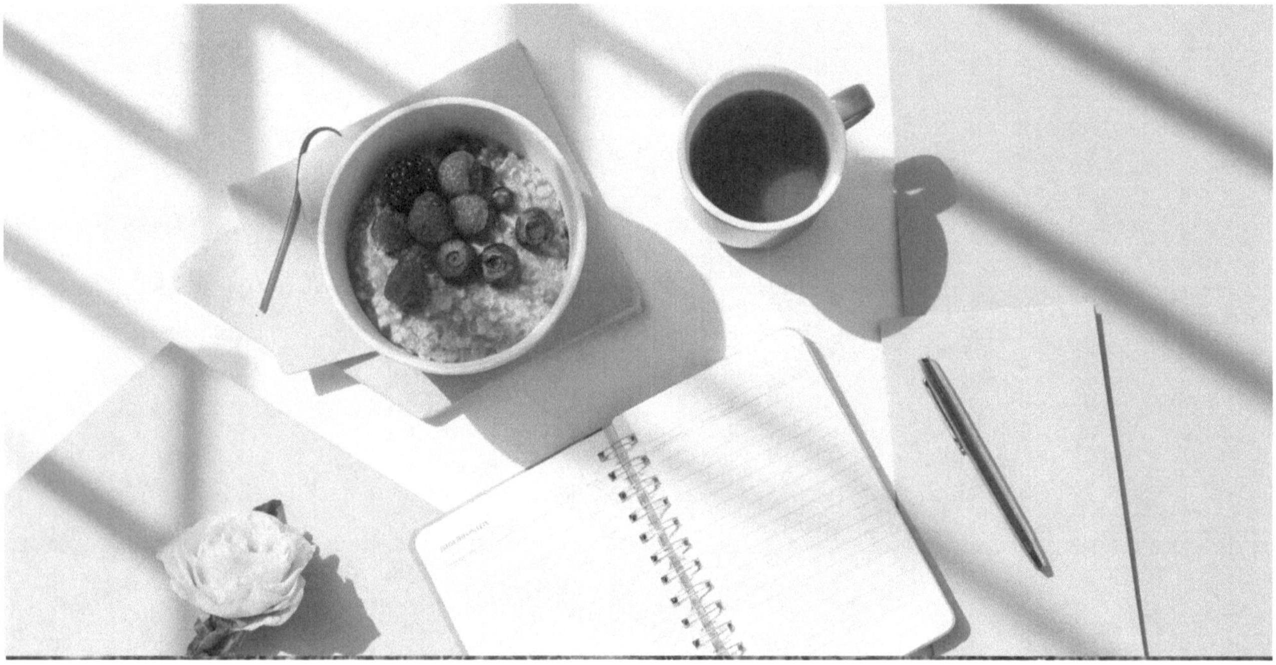

THE SCIENCE BEHIND THE DIET

The DASH diet didn't appear by accident. It was developed through extensive research by the U.S. National Heart, Lung, and Blood Institute, is a structured yet flexible eating plan proven to reduce hypertension. It emphasizes a variety of nutrient-rich foods—fruits, vegetables, whole grains, lean meats, nuts, and legumes—while discouraging sodium, red meats, and processed sugars. The focus on potassium, calcium, and magnesium helps stabilize blood pressure naturally, supporting cardiovascular and kidney function.

In clinical trials, individuals following the DASH plan experienced significant drops in both systolic and diastolic pressure, sometimes within two weeks. This effect was even stronger among those who reduced sodium below 2,300 mg per day. The diet also improves cholesterol balance and reduces inflammation, making it a powerful anti-inflammatory and heart smart eating plan.

This wasn't the result of pills or gimmicks. It was real, measurable improvement fueled by food choices. And what's even more remarkable is that participants didn't feel deprived. They ate satisfying meals that naturally balanced nutrients their bodies had been craving all along.

Unlike restrictive fads, the DASH method promotes variety and satisfaction. Seniors can enjoy flavorful salt-free cooking without compromising taste or nutrition. When paired with a Mediterranean diet influence—olive oil, fish, legumes, and fresh produce—it further enhances benefits for circulation and longevity. This combined approach also reduces risks of diabetes, stroke, and metabolic syndrome.

The Silent Killer

High blood pressure, or hypertension, is one of the most common yet silent conditions affecting millions of adults worldwide. It occurs when the force of blood pushing against artery walls remains consistently high, forcing the heart to work harder. Over time, this can lead to heart disease, kidney problems, stroke, and vision loss. For seniors, managing hypertension is crucial to maintaining independence and a high quality of life.

Several factors contribute to high blood pressure: genetics, sedentary lifestyles, processed foods, and chronic stress. Excess sodium and unhealthy fats can cause water retention, leading to swelling, fatigue, and elevated readings. The DASH diet was created as a solution to this growing health crisis, focusing on nutrient-rich foods that balance electrolytes, improve circulation, and support healthy heart function.

he DASH diet's nutrient balance helps manage hypertension, but its benefits extend beyond blood pressure. It boosts energy, supports digestion, and helps seniors maintain muscle and bone strength. Many find it easier to follow than calorie-counting plans because it focuses on food quality rather than deprivation.

Every recipe in this book reflects those principles—nutrient-dense, simple to prepare, and made with ingredients available at any grocery store. Caregivers will also find these meals easy to prepare and portion for seniors who prefer cooking for one or two. With practical meal prep guidance and clearly labeled grocery shopping lists, the plan promotes consistency and confidence in the kitchen. Ultimately, the DASH diet transforms food into medicine, providing a balanced approach that nourishes body and mind while managing hypertension naturally.

So what makes the DASH diet so effective?

For seniors, following the DASH diet offers life-changing rewards. It not only helps reduce blood pressure but also improves overall cardiovascular health, boosts energy, and promotes healthy aging. The plan's focus on nutrient-dense foods makes it ideal for maintaining muscle tone, bone strength, and mobility—key elements of independence in later years.

It focuses on restoring the natural balance of nutrients your body needs to thrive. One of the greatest advantages of this diet is its role in preventing heart failure, stroke, and atrial fibrillation.

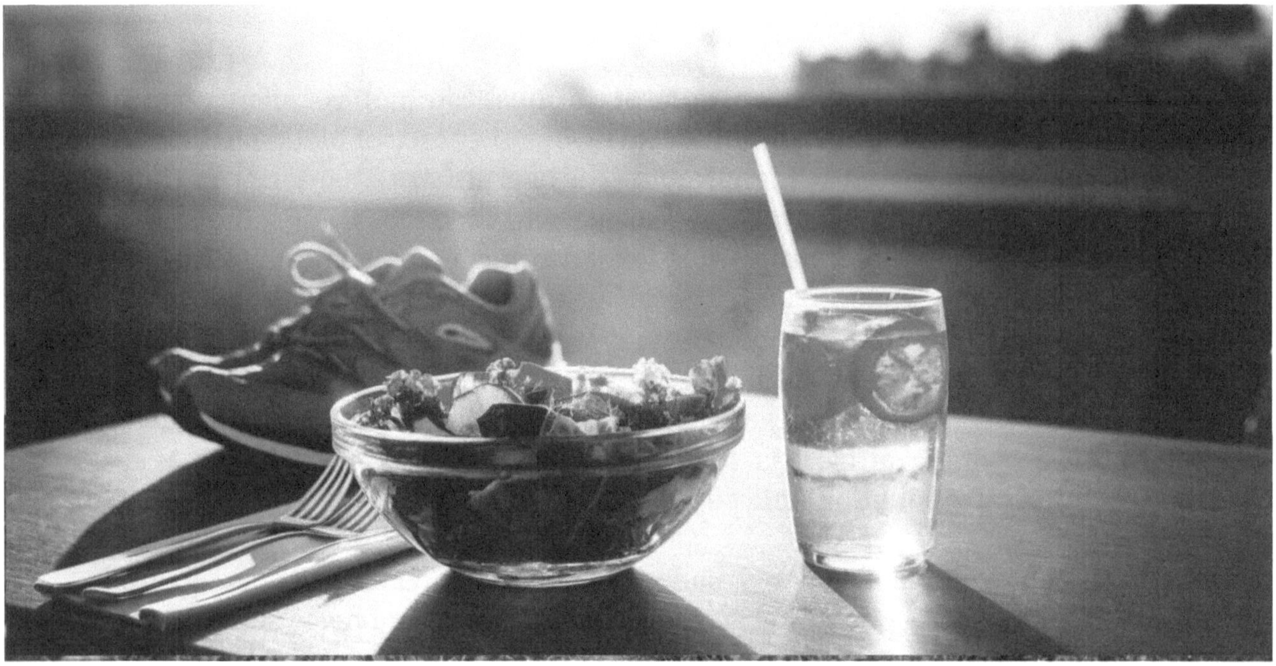

CORE PRINCIPLES

Here's how it works:

- Reducing salt helps decrease water retention and eases strain on your heart.
- Potassium helps your body release sodium through urine, balancing blood pressure.
- Fresh fruits, vegetables, whole grains, and lean proteins nourish your body while minimizing processed ingredients.

Why the DASH Diet Works for Seniors

- The balance of nutrients supports blood vessel elasticity and healthy circulation.
- Calcium, magnesium, and lean protein strengthen your frame and prevent weakness.
- Whole grains and plant-based meals sustain energy without blood sugar spikes.
- The natural antioxidants in fruits and vegetables fight chronic inflammation that contributes to heart disease and arthritis.
- Because meals are nutrient-dense and satisfying, you feel full longer and avoid overeating.

This is why the DASH diet is still considered one of the most effective heart-healthy eating plans worldwide. It's practical, flexible, and adaptable to your daily life. As a health expert, I've seen countless seniors regain control of their blood pressure, energy, and confidence through the DASH approach.

The power to transform your health has been on your plate all along. Now, it's time to use it.

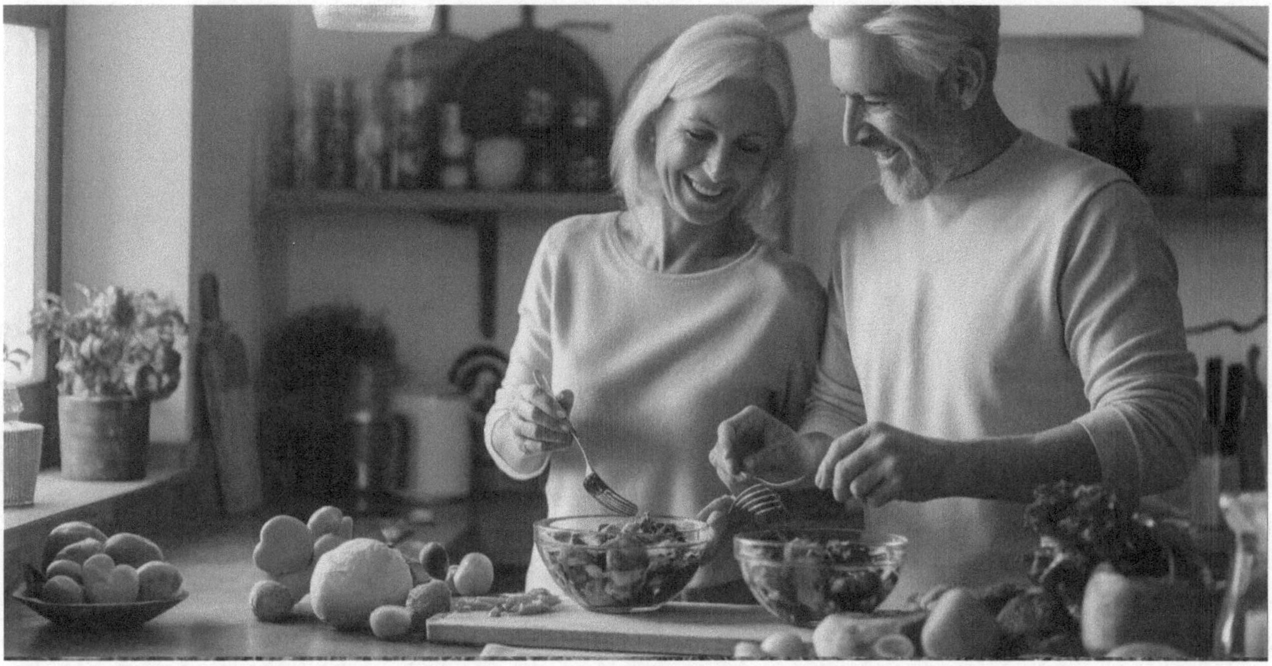

BENEFITS FOR OLDER ADULTS

When you follow the DASH diet, the first thing you'll notice isn't just a change in your blood pressure. It's how much better you feel overall. Your body starts to respond quickly to nourishment that supports your heart, bones, and mind. The food you eat becomes your energy source, not just another meal to get through.

Many seniors report improved circulation, less swelling in their hands and ankles, and even clearer thinking after just a few weeks. That's because your body works best when your heart doesn't have to struggle to push blood through your veins. The nutrients in DASH-friendly foods, like potassium, magnesium, and calcium, restore balance and ease the burden on your cardiovascular system.

You'll notice you can walk longer without feeling winded. You'll sleep better. You'll wake up refreshed instead of drained. These small improvements add up to something powerful—a renewed sense of control over your health.

The DASH diet also supports bone strength through calcium-rich foods like yogurt and leafy greens, helping reduce the risk of osteoporosis. Protein from fish, beans, and lean meats maintains muscle tone and supports recovery, especially if you're staying active. Beyond the physical benefits, you'll likely notice a positive shift in mood and motivation. When your body feels cared for, your confidence grows. That's the goal—to help you age with strength, clarity, and independence.

The DASH diet isn't about giving things up—it's about gaining something back: energy, vitality, and the freedom to enjoy life without the constant worry of health complications.

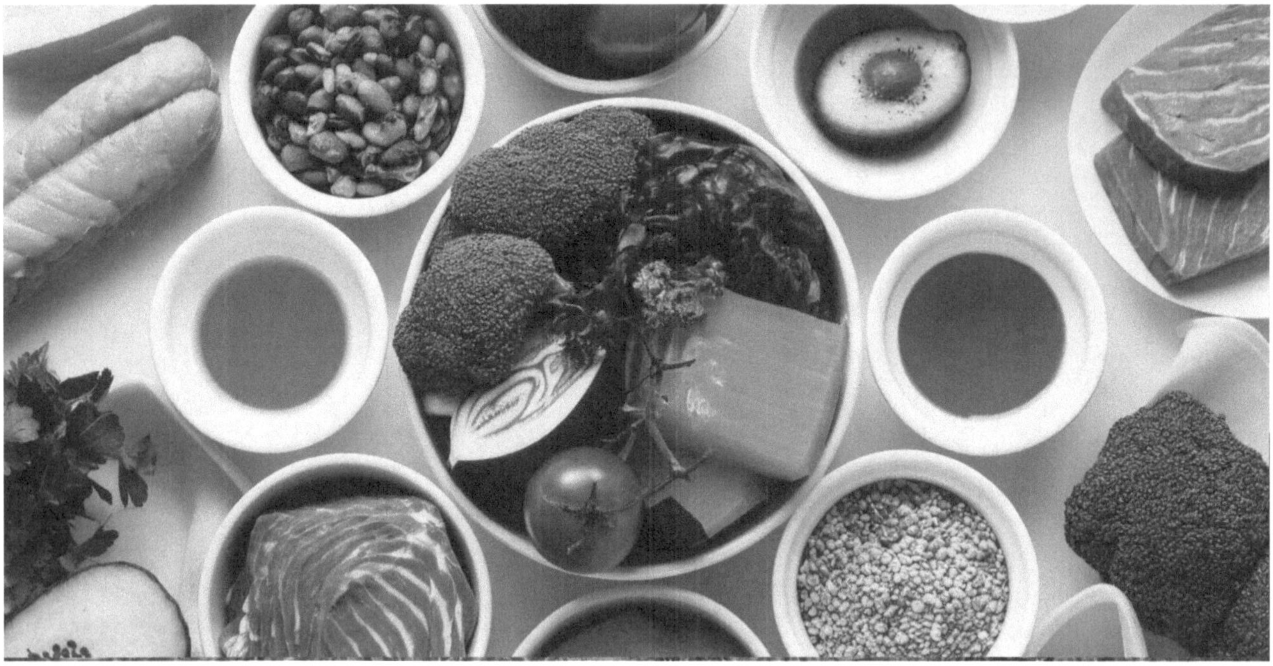

GETTING STARTED

Beginning the DASH diet can be one of the most rewarding steps toward a healthier, more active life. The plan encourages daily choices that lower blood pressure naturally and support long-term wellness. Before starting, it helps to understand the core food groups and portion guidelines that make up a balanced DASH plate. Each day, you'll aim for plenty of fruits and vegetables, whole grains, low-fat dairy, lean proteins, and small portions of healthy fats.

The heart healthy balance of these nutrients helps reduce sodium intake while providing potassium, calcium, and magnesium—minerals vital for heart function and bone strength. This guide makes it easy to follow whether you are new to the DASH plan or transitioning from another cardiac or Mediterranean diet. Simple instructions, clear measurements, and sample portion charts are included so you never feel lost.

Many seniors appreciate that the DASH plan allows flexibility for individual needs. If you are diabetic or managing cholesterol, there are diabetic friendly and low fat recipe options. Those following a soft food diet plan will also find easy-to-chew recipes that maintain flavor without heavy seasoning or salt. If you cook for one or two, each dish can be scaled down or refrigerated for later, ensuring minimal waste and maximum freshness.

Consistency is key. The 30-day meal plan in this cookbook is carefully designed to help seniors gradually adopt new habits without feeling deprived. Tracking progress in a blood pressure log book or food journal can keep motivation high. With time, you will notice not only reduced readings but also improved energy, better sleep, and a renewed sense of vitality. Starting the DASH diet is more than a nutrition shift—it's a lifestyle reset toward balance, independence, and heart smart living.

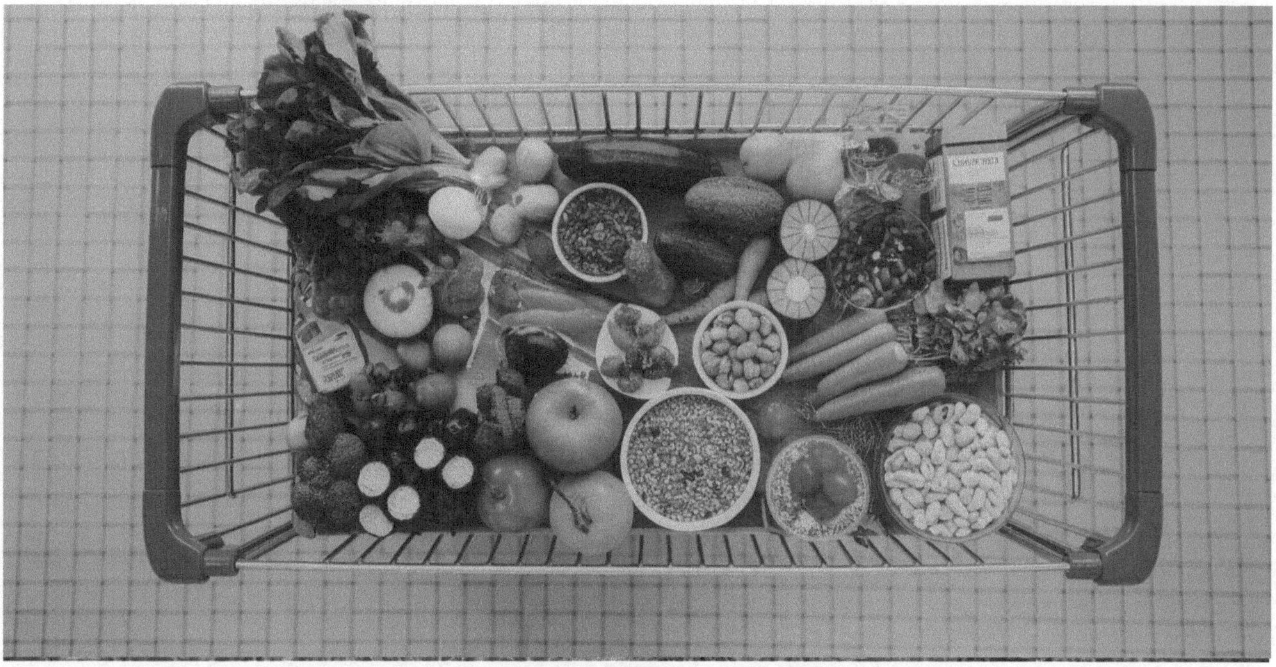

GROCERY SHOPPING FOR SUCCESS

A successful DASH journey begins at the grocery store. Smart shopping ensures your kitchen is stocked with everything needed for easy, low sodium recipes that promote wellness. Start by focusing on whole, unprocessed foods. Fresh fruits, vegetables, lean meats, beans, low-fat dairy, and whole grains should make up most of your cart. These items naturally provide the nutrients that lower blood pressure and reduce inflammation.

Reading food labels is crucial for managing sodium and fat intake. Look for "low sodium," "no salt added," or "heart healthy" indicators on packaging. Choose items with fewer than 140 mg of sodium per serving whenever possible. Avoid heavily processed foods, canned soups, or pre-seasoned mixes that often contain hidden salt and sugars. This careful selection supports better circulation and a strong cardiovascular system.

Creating a grocery list before shopping saves time and reduces stress. The lists included in this cookbook are designed for seniors, caregivers, or family members helping with meal prep for seniors. Items are grouped by food category and quantity, so shopping becomes simple and efficient. Many ingredients can also be bought frozen or pre-cut to save time in the kitchen without sacrificing nutrition.

As you adjust to the DASH lifestyle, experiment with colorful produce and whole grains to keep meals exciting. Sweet potatoes, avocados, quinoa, and spinach are all rich in minerals that promote healthy aging and reduce the risk of hypertension.

Consider this process part of your self-care routine. Each grocery trip is an investment in wellness, longevity, and energy. The more familiar you become with reading labels and making smart choices, the more natural heart smart cooking becomes. Over time, you'll notice your pantry evolving into a space filled with vitality, ready to support healthy eating habits and lifelong wellness for you and your loved ones.

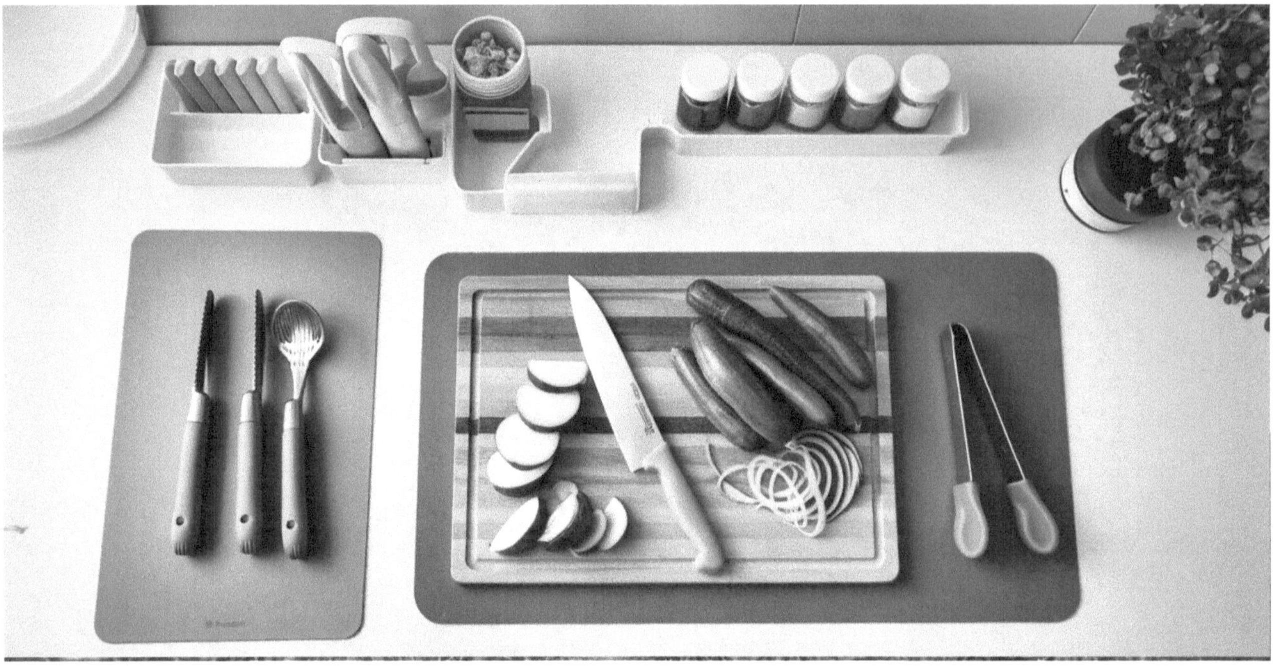

KITCHEN SAFETY AND COMFORT

A successful DASH journey begins at the grocery store. Smart shopping ensures your kitchen is stocked with everything needed for easy, low sodium recipes that promote wellness. Start by focusing on whole, unprocessed foods. Fresh fruits, vegetables, lean meats, beans, low-fat dairy, and whole grains should make up most of your cart. These items naturally provide the nutrients that lower blood pressure and reduce inflammation.

Reading food labels is crucial for managing sodium and fat intake. Look for "low sodium," "no salt added," or "heart healthy" indicators on packaging. Choose items with fewer than 140 mg of sodium per serving whenever possible. Avoid heavily processed foods, canned soups, or pre-seasoned mixes that often contain hidden salt and sugars. This careful selection supports better circulation and a strong cardiovascular system.

Creating a grocery list before shopping saves time and reduces stress. The lists included in this cookbook are designed for seniors, caregivers, or family members helping with meal prep for seniors. Items are grouped by food category and quantity, so shopping becomes simple and efficient. Many ingredients can also be bought frozen or pre-cut to save time in the kitchen without sacrificing nutrition.

As you adjust to the DASH lifestyle, experiment with colorful produce and whole grains to keep meals exciting. Sweet potatoes, avocados, quinoa, and spinach are all rich in minerals that promote healthy aging and reduce the risk of hypertension.

Consider this process part of your self-care routine. Each grocery trip is an investment in wellness, longevity, and energy. The more familiar you become with reading labels and making smart choices, the more natural heart smart cooking becomes. Over time, you'll notice your pantry evolving into a space filled with vitality, ready to support healthy eating habits and lifelong wellness for you and your loved ones.

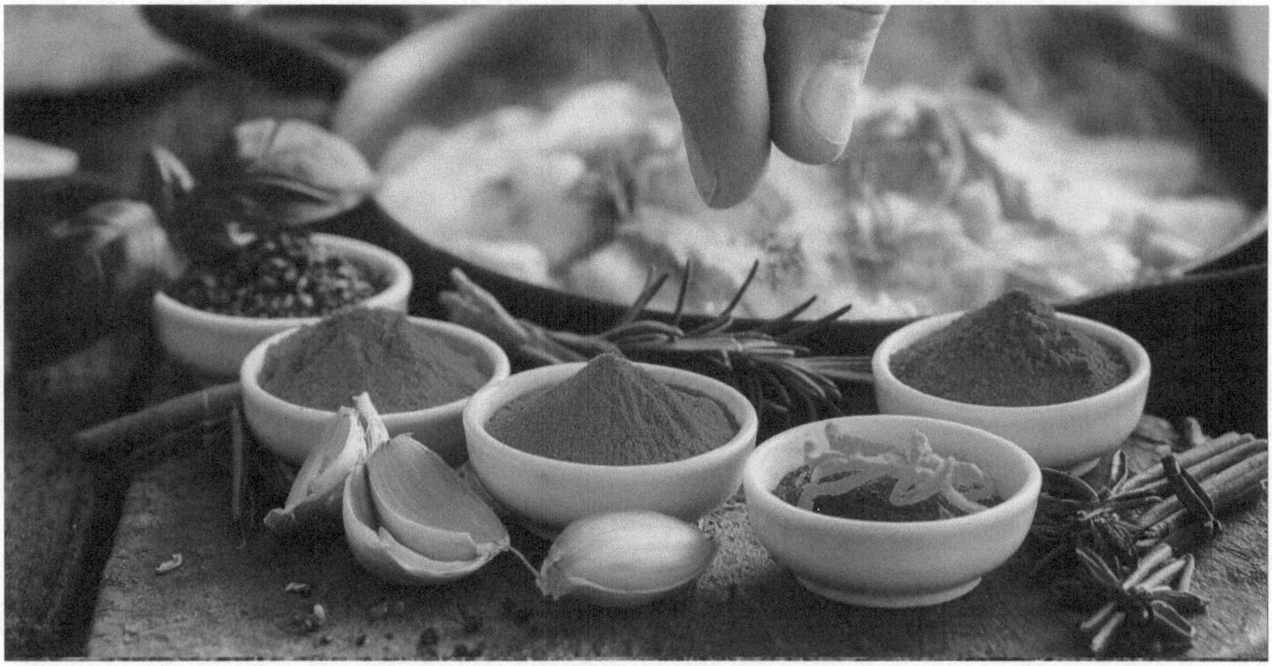

FLAVOR WITHOUT SALT

One of the greatest misconceptions about heart healthy cooking is that reducing salt means sacrificing flavor. The DASH diet proves the opposite. By learning how to season meals naturally, you can enjoy vibrant, satisfying dishes while lowering blood pressure and supporting overall health.

Flavorful salt-free cooking begins with herbs, spices, and natural acids. Garlic, onion, lemon, vinegar, pepper, and fresh herbs like rosemary or basil enhance taste without adding sodium. Mixing herbs with citrus or olive oil creates aromatic dressings and marinades that elevate vegetables, poultry, and fish. This simple technique allows seniors to enjoy gourmet flavors at home without extra effort.

Spice blends such as paprika, cumin, turmeric, and chili powder not only add variety but also provide anti-inflammatory benefits. Using them regularly can reduce water retention and promote better circulation. Try pairing herbs and spices by cuisine type—for example, oregano and thyme for Mediterranean meals or ginger and cilantro for Asian-inspired dishes.

Another trick is to balance texture and aroma. Roasting vegetables brings out their natural sweetness, while using vinegar or balsamic glazes adds tangy brightness. Low sodium broths, tomato purees, or beans can add depth to soups and stews without added salt.

This cookbook includes a flavor guide to inspire experimentation. Each recipe is tested for taste, ensuring you never feel deprived. With these methods, even simple meals for one or two can become exciting and satisfying. Ultimately, the goal is not to remove flavor but to rediscover it naturally.

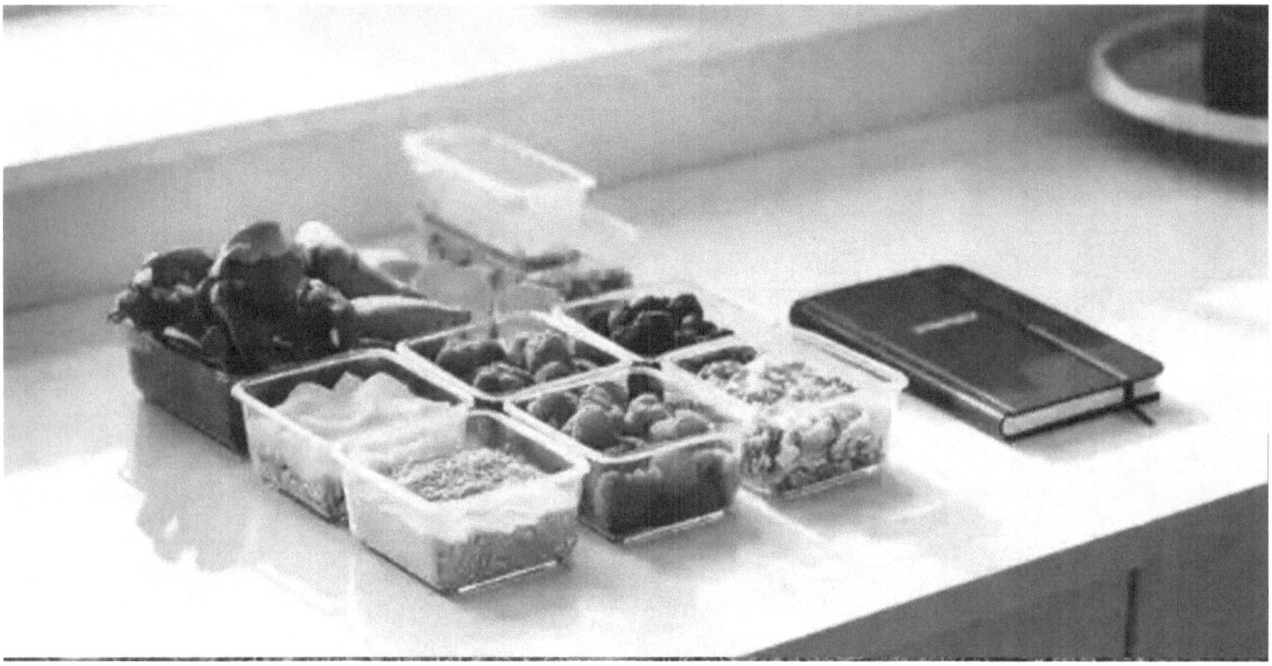

MEAL PREP MADE SIMPLE

Meal preparation is one of the most effective ways for seniors to stay consistent with the DASH diet. By setting aside time each week to plan and cook, you can lower blood pressure naturally, reduce stress, and make heart healthy eating easier than ever.

Why Meal Prep Matters

- Saves time and energy – No need to cook from scratch daily.
- Supports portion control – Prevents overeating and helps maintain healthy weight.
- Reduces sodium intake – Homemade meals mean full control of salt levels.
- Boosts vitality – Nutrient-rich, balanced meals provide steady energy.
- Improves heart function – Regularly eating DASH-approved foods supports circulation and reduces cholesterol.

For older adults, meal prep means freedom from constant kitchen work and more time for family, hobbies, or relaxation.

Step 1: Plan Your Week

Start with your 30-day DASH meal plan from this cookbook. Choose which meals you'll repeat or batch cook. Then create a weekly grocery list focusing on:

Food Group	DASH-Approved Examples	Benefits
Fruits & Vegetables	Spinach, berries, bananas, carrots, broccoli	High in potassium and antioxidants
Whole Grains	Oats, brown rice, quinoa, whole wheat pasta	Stabilize blood sugar and improve digestion
Lean Proteins	Chicken, turkey, salmon, beans, tofu	Support muscle and heart health
Low-Fat Dairy	Skim milk, yogurt, cottage cheese	Calcium for strong bones
Healthy Fats	Olive oil, avocado, nuts	Reduce inflammation and improve cholesterol

When shopping, read labels carefully:

- Choose "low sodium" or "no salt added" items.
- Limit anything with over 140 mg sodium per serving.
- Avoid canned soups, processed meats, and instant noodles.

Step 2: Batch Cook and Store

Pick one or two days a week to cook in larger batches. Examples:

- Sunday: Prepare two soups, a grain base (quinoa or brown rice), and roasted vegetables.
- Wednesday: Cook a protein like chicken or salmon and prepare two soft food diet options for variety.

Store meals in labeled containers.

Storage Method	Shelf Life	Tips
Refrigerator	3–4 days	Use clear containers to see contents easily.
Freezer	Up to 3 months	Label with name and date for safety.

Quick tip:
For caregivers, pre-labeled meals make it simple to reheat and serve without confusion.

Step 3: Flavor Without Salt

Add taste and excitement to your meals naturally:

- Herbs: Basil, oregano, rosemary, thyme
- Spices: Paprika, cumin, turmeric, pepper
- Acidic Additions: Lemon juice, lime, vinegar
- Healthy Fats: Olive oil, tahini, avocado

These provide anti-inflammatory benefits, improve circulation, and keep meals satisfying without sodium.

Step 4: Keep Track and Stay Motivated

Use a Blood Pressure Log Book or meal tracker to record what you eat and how you feel.

You may notice:

- Higher energy levels
- Better digestion
- Improved sleep
- More stable blood pressure readings

Meal Prep Example Day

Meal	Example	Notes
Breakfast	Oatmeal with banana and cinnamon	Easy to make ahead, low sodium
Lunch	Quinoa bowl with chickpeas and spinach	Great for batch cooking
Dinner	Baked salmon, sweet potatoes and green beans	Heart healthy, anti-inflammatory

Final Thoughts

Meal prep for seniors isn't just about convenience—it's about empowerment. Whether you're cooking for one, sharing with a partner, or gifting meals to a loved one, planning ahead ensures every plate supports healthy aging and heart wellness.

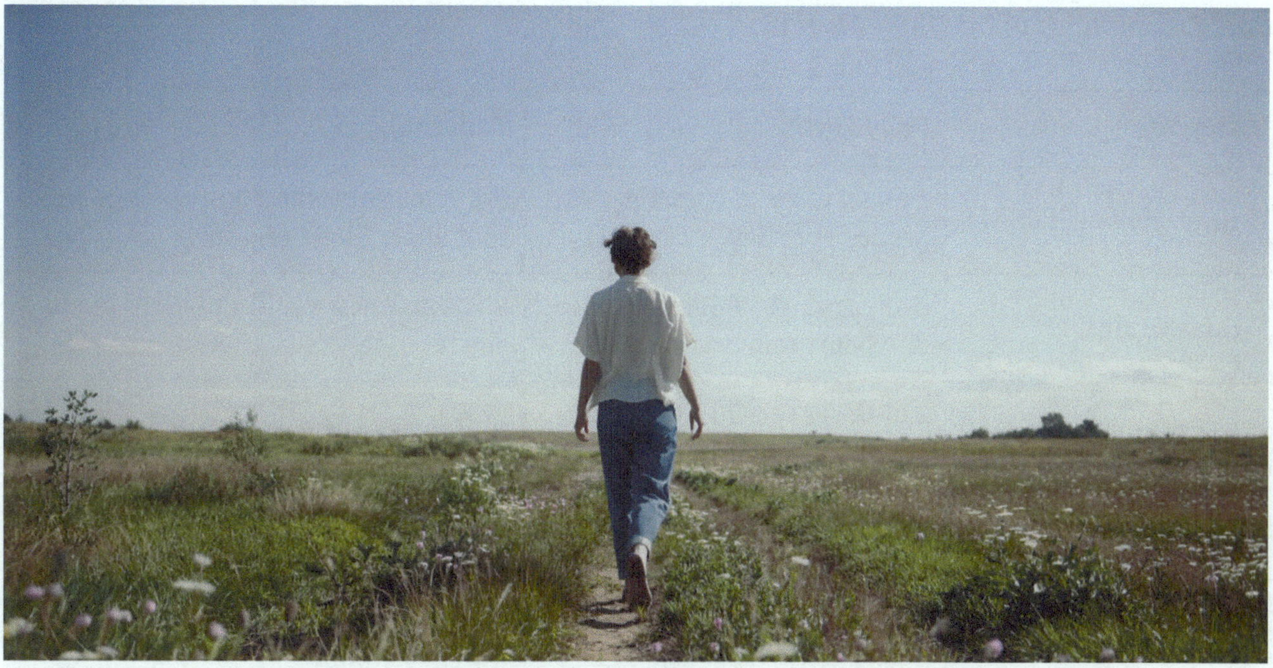

THE 30-DAY DASH MEAL PLAN OVERVIEW

The 30-Day DASH Meal Plan in this cookbook is designed to make healthy eating effortless and enjoyable for seniors. It brings together simplicity, flavor, and science-backed nutrition to help you reduce blood pressure naturally, maintain steady energy levels, and promote overall wellness. Each week builds upon the previous one, allowing your body to adjust to new eating habits while keeping meals satisfying and practical.

This plan includes breakfast, lunch, and dinner ideas for every day, featuring low sodium, heart healthy recipes that are easy to follow and require only simple ingredients. The structure accommodates different needs—whether you're cooking for one or two, following a soft food diet, or managing conditions like diabetes, high cholesterol, or atrial fibrillation. The variety ensures that you never get bored, while the balanced portions help you manage hypertension, weight, and energy levels effectively.

Sample One-Day Menu

Meal	Example	Why It Works
Breakfast	Green Morning Smoothie with spinach, banana, and low-fat yogurt	High in potassium and calcium for better heart rhythm
Lunch	Blackened Shrimp and Avocado Tacos	Provides lean protein and healthy fats without excess sodium
Dinner	Chicken Cutlets with Sun-Dried Tomato Sauce and Steamed Vegetables	Balanced meal with low cholesterol and rich flavor

Core Components of the DASH Meal Plan

Category	Daily Focus	Benefits
Fruits and Vegetables	4–5 servings of colorful produce per day	Provides potassium and antioxidants that lower blood pressure
Whole Grains	6–8 servings of oatmeal, rice, or whole grain bread	Sustains energy and stabilizes blood sugar
Lean Proteins	2 or fewer servings of poultry, fish, beans, or tofu	Builds muscle, reduces cholesterol
Low-Fat Dairy	2–3 servings of yogurt, milk, or cheese	Strengthens bones and supports metabolism
Healthy Fats	Limited to 2–3 servings of olive oil, nuts, or seeds	Improves circulation and reduces inflammation
Sodium Intake	Under 2,300 mg daily (1 teaspoon of salt)	Helps regulate fluid balance and manage hypertension
Sweets	3 or fewer servings per week	Keeps sugar intake minimal while allowing enjoyment

Week 1 – Fresh Start for Your Heart

The first week focuses on gradual adjustments and creating a foundation for healthy living. Rather than changing everything overnight, you'll begin by reducing sodium and adding more fresh produce and whole grains to your meals. Drink plenty of water and avoid carbonated or sugary drinks.

Goals for Week 1:

- Replace processed snacks with fruits or nuts.
- Use herbs, lemon, or vinegar instead of salt.
- Eat three balanced meals a day with one healthy snack.
- Keep sodium below 2,300 mg daily.

Example Meal	Description
Breakfast	Oatmeal with bananas and cinnamon (fiber-rich and satisfying)
Lunch	Grilled chicken salad with olive oil and balsamic vinegar
Dinner	Baked salmon with steamed vegetables and brown rice

Week 2 – Boosting Energy and Confidence

In Week 2, your body begins adapting to the DASH lifestyle. You'll feel more energized, thanks to balanced meals that stabilize blood sugar and improve circulation. Focus on variety and flavor—introduce colorful vegetables, lean proteins, and a mix of healthy fats.

Goals for Week 2:

- Try one new fruit or vegetable daily. Also include a serving of beans, lentils, or quinoa.
- Reduce refined grains and switch to whole grain pasta or bread.
- Add light physical activity such as walking or stretching.

You'll start noticing improved digestion, higher stamina, and fewer cravings for salty or sugary foods.

Example Meal	Description
Breakfast	Greek yogurt with berries and flaxseeds
Lunch	Quinoa and veggie bowl with chickpeas
Dinner	Chicken and mushroom stir-fry with brown rice

Week 3 – Strengthening Heart and Mind

By Week 3, your routine becomes second nature. The focus now shifts to strengthening your heart and sharpening mental clarity. The DASH plan's anti-inflammatory meals—rich in omega-3 fats, antioxidants, and minerals—work to reduce swelling, promote better circulation, and support brain function.

Goals for Week 3:

- Emphasize fish, nuts, and leafy greens.
- Limit red meat and avoid fried foods entirely.
- Practice mindful eating: slow down and enjoy each meal.

This week strengthens heart rhythm, improves sleep, and enhances energy throughout the day, leading to an overall sense of vitality.

Example Meal	Description
Breakfast	Vegetable omelet with spinach and mushrooms
Lunch	Tuna and avocado wrap with side salad
Dinner	Baked chicken with roasted Brussels sprouts and sweet potatoes

Week 4 – Building Long-Term Healthy Habits

The final week helps you transition from a structured plan to a sustainable lifestyle. By now, your taste buds have adjusted to natural flavors, and your body feels lighter and more balanced. This stage focuses on maintaining motivation, portion control, and continued variety in meals.

Goals for Week 4:

- Focus on portion sizes—avoid overeating even healthy foods.
- Treat yourself occasionally, but stay mindful.
- Encourage family participation for ongoing support.

By the end of Week 4, you've established strong habits for managing hypertension, boosting energy, and maintaining heart smart nutrition. The DASH diet becomes not just a 30-day plan, but a lifelong commitment to healthy aging and vitality.

Example Meal	Description
Breakfast	Smoothie with spinach, apple, and low-fat yogurt
Lunch	Lentil soup with whole grain toast
Dinner	Grilled shrimp with vegetables and quinoa

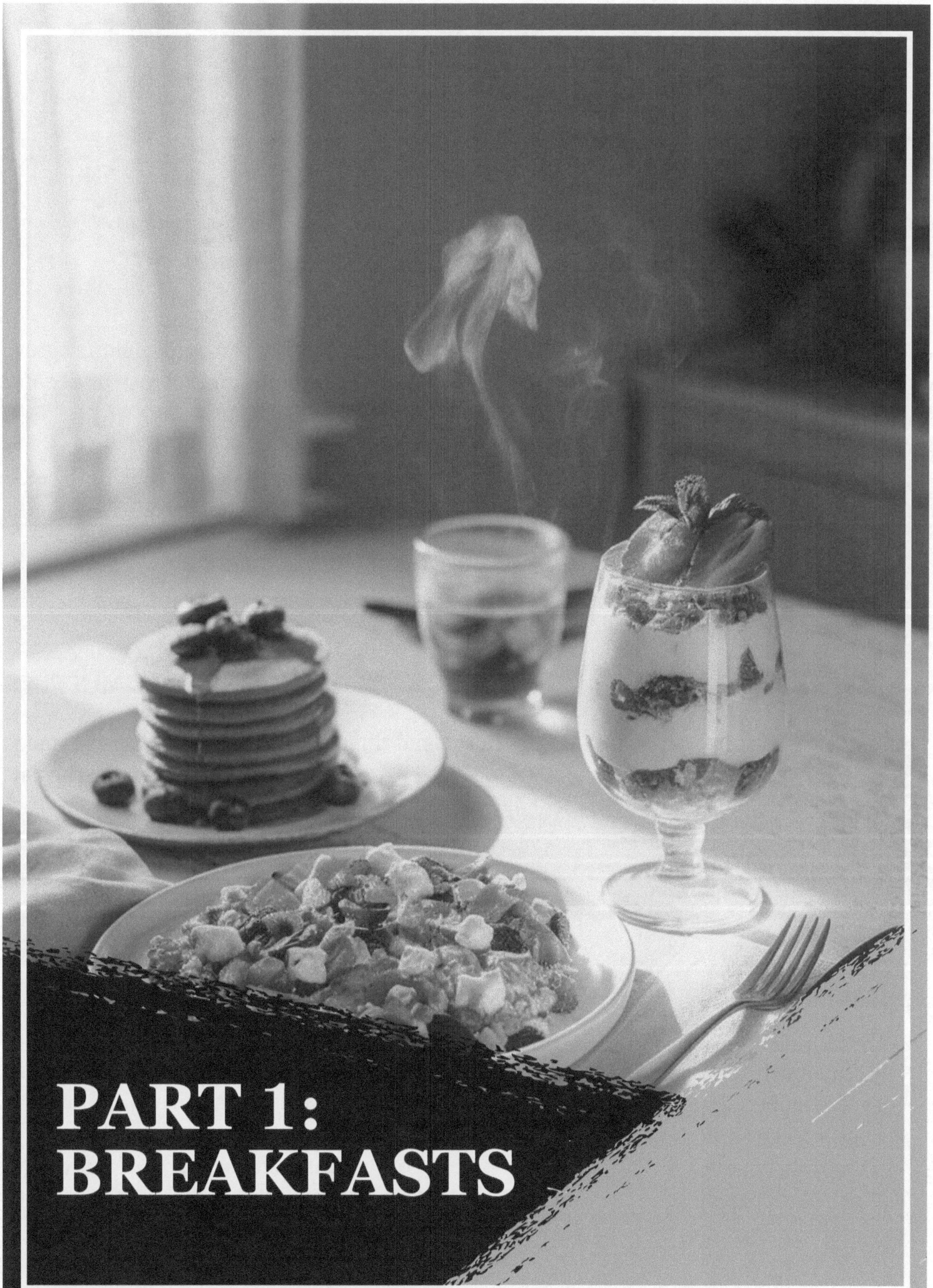

PART 1: BREAKFASTS

1. VEGETABLE AND FETA CHEESE SCRAMBLE

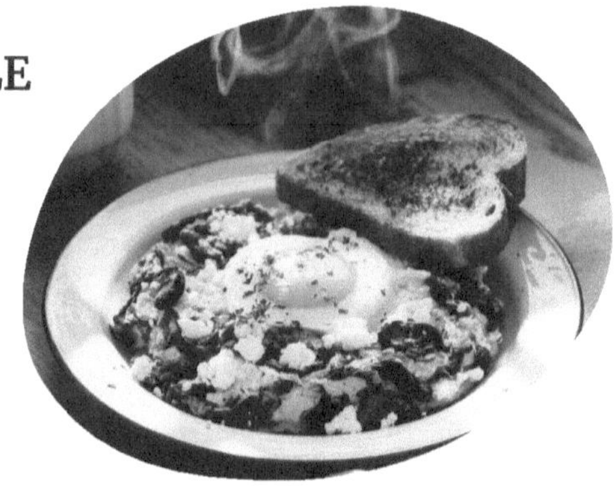

Light, fluffy, and filled with fresh greens for a balanced start to the day.

Nutrition (per serving): 165 calories, 10g protein, 10g fat, 5g carbs, 220mg sodium.

INGREDIENTS

- Cooking spray
- ½ cup mushrooms, sliced
- 1 cup chopped spinach
- 1 egg + 2 egg whites
- 2 tbsp feta cheese
- Pinch black pepper

INSTRUCTIONS

- Heat a non-stick pan with cooking spray.
- Sauté mushrooms and spinach until soft.
- In a bowl, whisk egg and egg whites.
- Stir in feta and pepper.
- Pour mixture into skillet; cook until set.
- Serve warm with whole-grain toast.

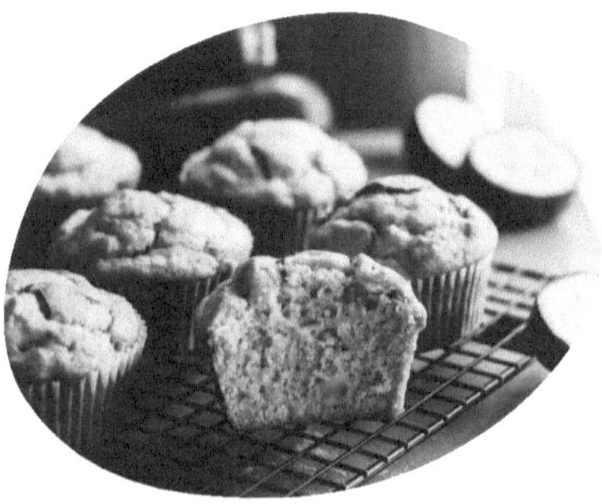

2. ZUCCHINI MIX MUFFINS

Light, fluffy, and filled with fresh greens for a balanced start to the day.

Nutrition (per serving):
Calories: ~340 |
Protein: 26 g |
Carbs: 28 g | Fat: 14 g | Sodium: 130 mg

INGREDIENTS

- Cooking spray
- ½ cup mushrooms, sliced
- 1 cup chopped spinach
- 1 egg + 2 egg whites
- 2 tbsp feta cheese
- Pinch black pepper

INSTRUCTIONS

- Heat a non-stick pan with cooking spray.
- Sauté mushrooms and spinach until soft.
- In a bowl, whisk egg and egg whites.
- Stir in feta and pepper.
- Pour mixture into skillet; cook until set.
- Serve warm with whole-grain toast.

3. EASY CHIVE OMELET

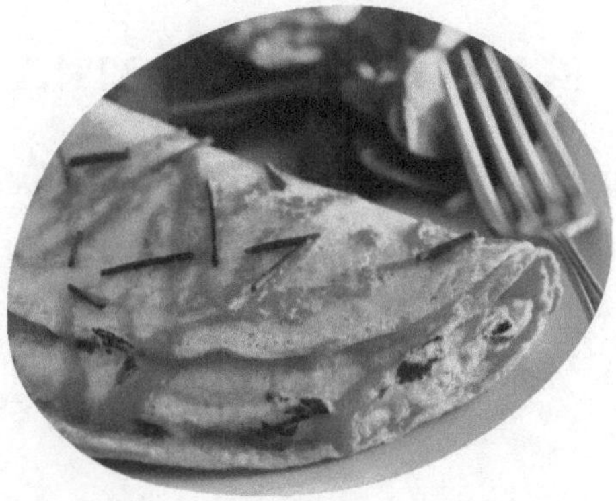

Fluffy, herb-filled, and naturally low in sodium.

Nutrition: 180 kcal, 15g protein, 10g fat, 4g carbs, 190mg sodium

INGREDIENTS

- 4 eggs
- 2 tbsp chopped chives
- 1/4 tsp salt
- Dash pepper
- 1/4 cup low-fat cheddar
- 1 cup baby spinach

INSTRUCTIONS

- Whisk eggs with salt, pepper, and chives.
- Heat a non-stick skillet and pour in mixture.
- Cook gently over medium heat.
- Add spinach and cheese as it sets.
- Fold and cook for one minute.
- Serve warm.

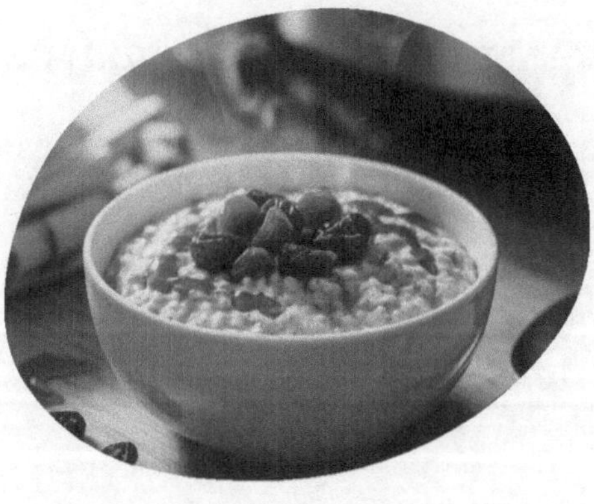

4. OATMEAL REST

Warm, creamy oats rich in fiber and natural sweetness.

Nutrition: 210 kcal, 8g protein, 3g fat, 38g carbs, 95mg sodium

INGREDIENTS

- 3 cups skim milk
- 2 cups water
- 2 cups steel-cut oats
- 1/4 cup raisins
- 1/4 cup dried cherries
- 1/4 tsp cinnamon
- 1 tsp honey

INSTRUCTIONS

- Combine all ingredients in a slow cooker.
- Stir and cover with lid.
- Cook on low for 8–9 hours.
- Stir before serving and drizzle with honey.

5. FRUIT GREEN SMOOTHIE

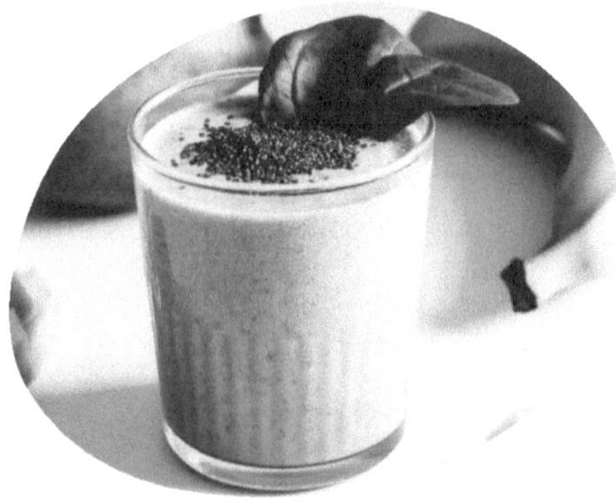

Refreshing, fiber-rich, and perfect for a quick breakfast.

Nutrition: 180 kcal, 7g protein, 3g fat, 33g carbs, 60mg sodium

INGREDIENTS

- 1 banana
- 1 cup spinach
- ½ cup skim milk
- ½ cup frozen mango
- ¼ cup yogurt
- 1 tbsp oats

INSTRUCTIONS

- Blend oats and milk for 15 seconds.
- Add spinach, banana, yogurt, and mango.
- Blend until smooth and creamy.
- Serve immediately, chilled.

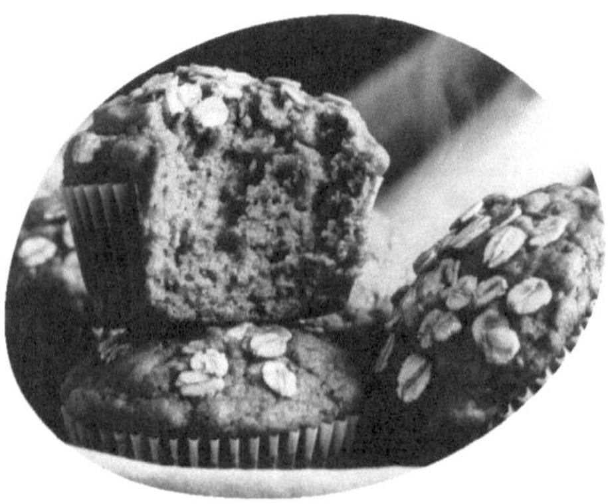

6. BANANA AND OATS MUFFINS

Naturally sweet and high in fiber for steady energy.

Nutrition: 165 kcal, 4g protein, 3g fat, 31g carbs, 110mg sodium

INGREDIENTS

- 1 cup whole wheat flour
- 1 cup oats
- 1 tsp baking soda
- 2 tbsp ground flaxseed
- 3 bananas, mashed
- ½ cup Greek yogurt
- ¼ cup unsweetened applesauce

INSTRUCTIONS

- Preheat oven to 355°F.
- Mix flour, oats, soda, and flaxseed.
- Blend bananas, yogurt, and applesauce.
- Combine wet and dry mixtures.
- Fill muffin cups and bake for 25 minutes.

7. SPICY TOMATO AND HERB BAKED EGGS

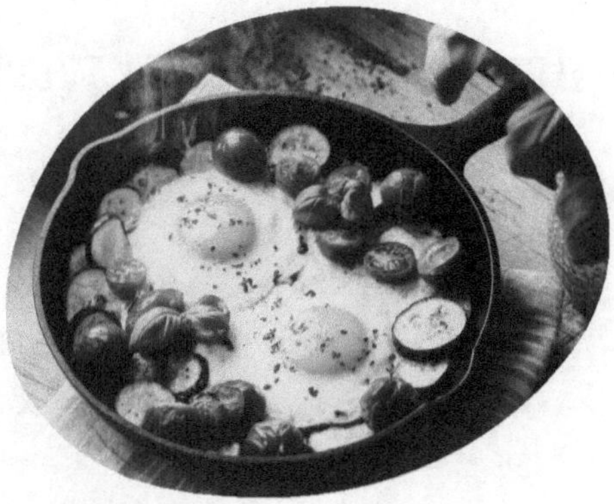

Simple, low-sodium, and bursting with Mediterranean flavor.

Nutrition: 170 kcal, 9g protein, 11g fat, 8g carbs, 130mg sodium

INGREDIENTS

- 1 tbsp olive oil
- 1 zucchini, diced
- 1 cup cherry tomatoes, halved
- 1 garlic clove, minced
- 2 eggs
- Fresh basil leaves

INSTRUCTIONS

- Heat olive oil in skillet.
- Add zucchini and cook for 5 minutes.
- Toss in tomatoes and garlic.
- Crack eggs into mixture and cover.
- Cook until whites are firm.
- Garnish with basil.

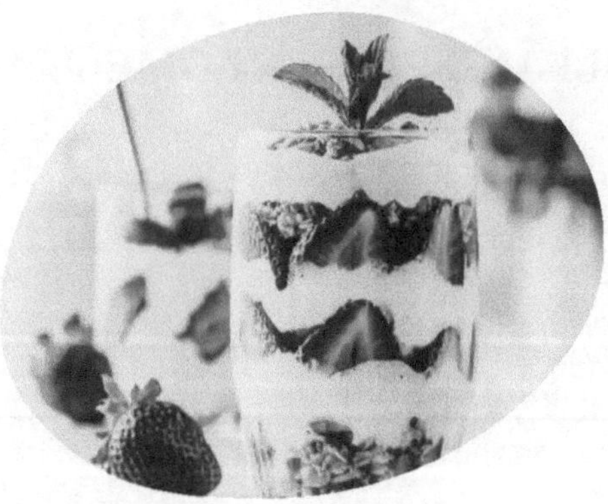

8. STRAWBERRY AND YOGURT PARFAIT

Sweet, light, and high in calcium for healthy bones.

Nutrition: 145 kcal, 7g protein, 3g fat, 22g carbs, 85mg sodium

INGREDIENTS

- ½ cup diced strawberries
- ½ cup low-fat vanilla yogurt
- 2 tbsp low-fat granola
- 1 mint sprig

INSTRUCTIONS

- Layer half the strawberries in a glass.
- Add yogurt, then the rest of the fruit.
- Top with granola and mint.
- Serve chilled.

9. BREAKFAST BARLEY WITH BANANA & HONEY

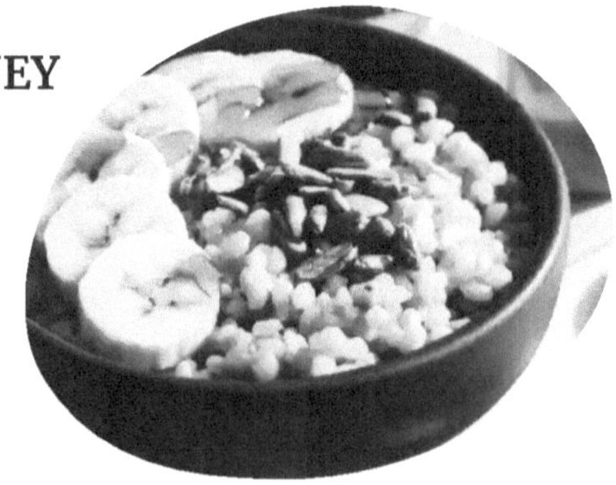

Hearty, simple, and naturally sweetened.

Nutrition: 190 kcal, 5g protein, 4g fat, 35g carbs, 70mg sodium

INGREDIENTS

- ½ cup quick-cooking barley
- 1 banana, sliced
- 1 tsp honey
- 1 tbsp sunflower seeds
- ¾ cup water

INSTRUCTIONS

- Boil barley in water for six minutes.
- Let stand for two minutes.
- Stir in banana and honey.
- Top with sunflower seeds and serve warm.

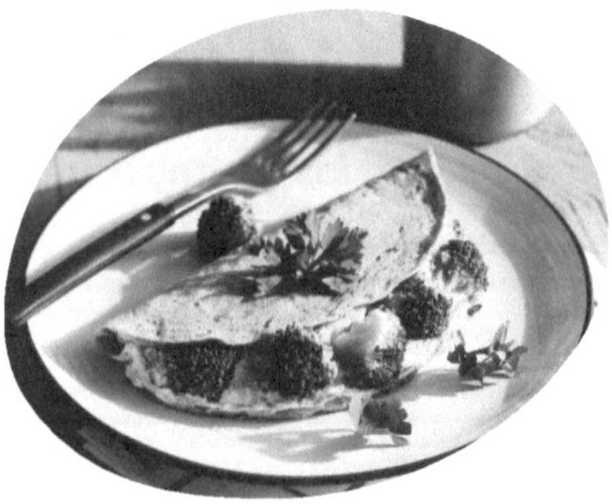

10. BROCCOLI AND PARSLEY OMELET

A light and nutrient-rich dish for steady morning energy.

Nutrition: 200 kcal, 13g protein, 13g fat, 4g carbs, 180mg sodium

INGREDIENTS

- 4 eggs
- ½ tsp salt
- ¼ tsp pepper
- 1 tbsp olive oil
- 1 cup chopped broccoli
- 1 tbsp parsley

INSTRUCTIONS

- Whisk eggs with salt and pepper.
- Heat olive oil in skillet.
- Add broccoli and sauté briefly.
- Pour in eggs and cook both sides.
- Top with parsley and serve.

11. CINNAMON FLAVORED APPLE GRANOLA

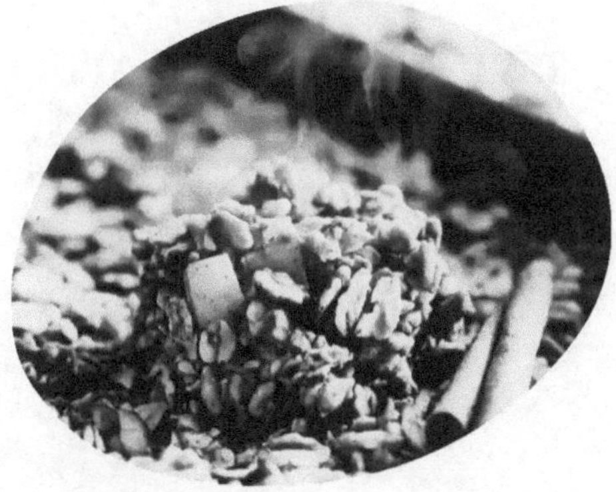

Crunchy, aromatic, and perfect for yogurt or snacking.

Nutrition: 210 kcal, 4g protein, 8g fat, 31g carbs, 75mg sodium

INGREDIENTS

- 3 cups oats
- ½ cup chopped walnuts
- ¼ cup applesauce
- ¼ cup honey
- 2 tbsp brown sugar
- 1 tsp cinnamon
- 1 cup dried apple pieces

INSTRUCTIONS

- Mix oats, nuts, and cinnamon in bowl.
- Warm applesauce, sugar, and honey.
- Pour over oat mixture and stir.
- Spread on tray and bake at 250°F for 90 minutes.
- Cool and add dried apples.

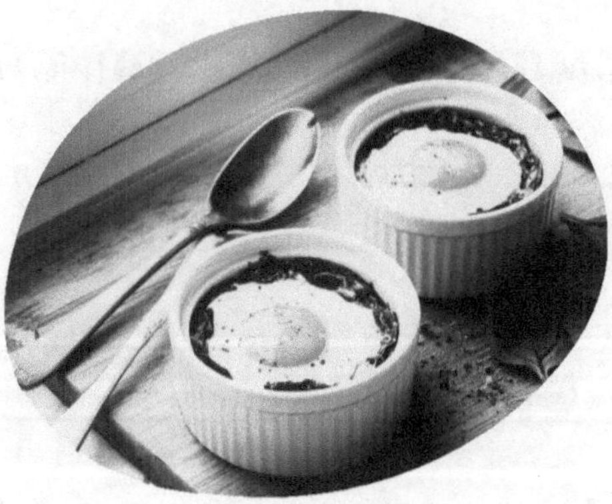

12. SPINACH AND EGGS FLORENTINE

Protein-packed, quick, and rich in iron.

Nutrition: 160 kcal, 10g protein, 11g fat, 3g carbs, 150mg sodium

INGREDIENTS

- 6 oz chopped spinach
- 4 eggs
- 2 tbsp olive oil
- 1 tsp seasoning

INSTRUCTIONS

- Preheat oven to 350°F.
- Place spinach in ramekins and make a small well.
- Crack an egg into each well.
- Drizzle olive oil and season lightly.
- Bake for eight minutes until eggs are set.

13. TWIN BERRY PARFAIT

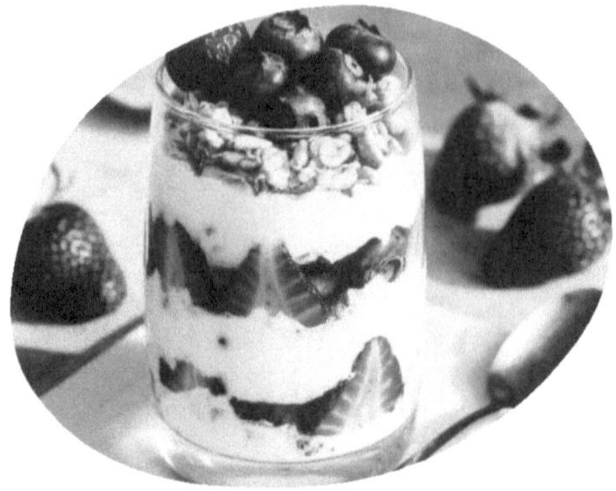

A sweet, antioxidant-rich layered breakfast.

Nutrition: 155 kcal, 6g protein, 2g fat, 28g carbs, 80mg sodium

INGREDIENTS

- 1 cup strawberries
- 1 cup blueberries
- 1 cup vanilla yogurt
- 2 tbsp granola

INSTRUCTIONS

- Add a layer of yogurt to a glass.
- Top with berries and granola.
- Repeat until glass is filled.
- Serve chilled.

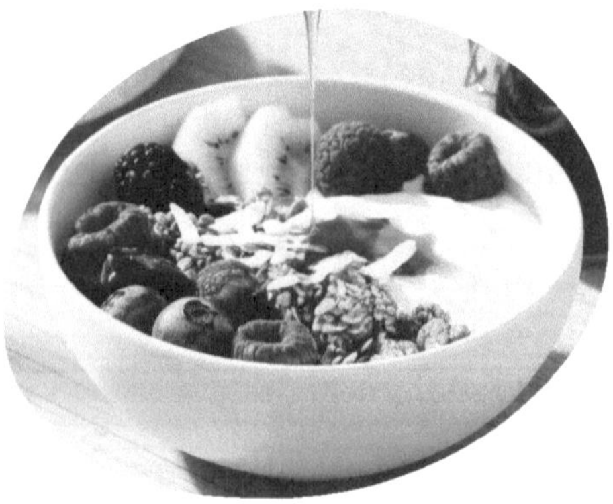

14. EARLY MORNING FRUIT CRUNCH

A bright, fruity start packed with fiber and hydration.

Nutrition: 175 kcal, 5g protein, 4g fat, 31g carbs, 65mg sodium

INGREDIENTS

- 2 cups mixed fruit
- 1 cup vanilla yogurt
- 1 tbsp honey
- ¼ cup granola
- 2 tbsp shredded coconut

INSTRUCTIONS

- Arrange fruit in bowls.
- Spoon yogurt on top.
- Drizzle with honey.
- Sprinkle granola and coconut before serving.

15. EASY EGG SANDWICH

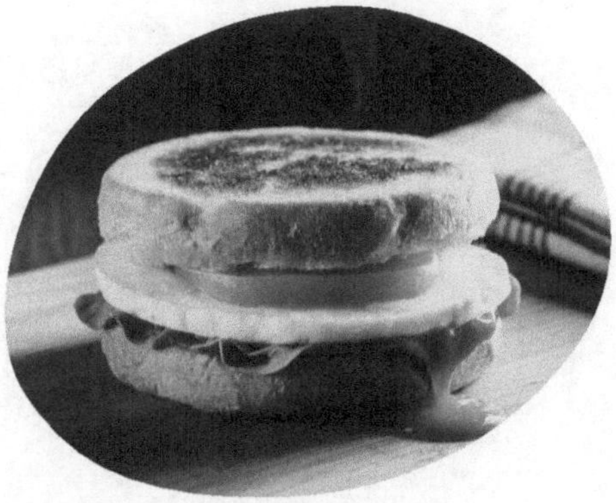

Protein-packed and ready in minutes. Ideal for busy mornings.

Nutrition: 210 kcal, 12g protein, 8g fat, 22g carbs, 230mg sodium

INGREDIENTS

- 1 whole-wheat English muffin
- 1 egg
- 1 slice low-fat cheese
- 1 tsp apricot preserve
- Cooking spray

INSTRUCTIONS

- Spray skillet and cook egg both sides.
- Toast muffin and spread preserve.
- Add cheese and cooked egg.
- Top with remaining muffin half and serve warm.

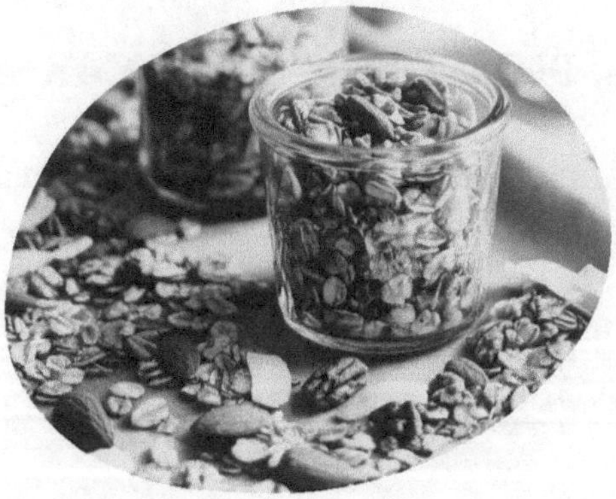

16. HONEY MIXED OATS GRANOLA

Crunchy, nutty, and naturally sweetened. Perfect for heart-healthy mornings.

Nutrition: 220 kcal, 5g protein, 9g fat, 31g carbs, 65mg sodium

INGREDIENTS

- 1/4 cup canola oil
- 4 tbsp honey
- 1 1/2 tsp vanilla extract
- 6 cups rolled oats
- 1 cup slivered almonds
- 1/2 cup unsweetened coconut
- 3/4 cup chopped walnuts
- 1 cup raisins

INSTRUCTIONS

- Preheat oven to 325°F.
- Warm oil, honey, and vanilla in a pan.
- Mix oats, almonds, coconut, and walnuts in a bowl.
- Pour warm mixture over oats and stir until coated.
- Bake on a parchment-lined tray for 25 minutes, stirring halfway.
- Cool, add raisins, and store airtight.

17. BROCCOLI, ONION AND CARROT OMELET

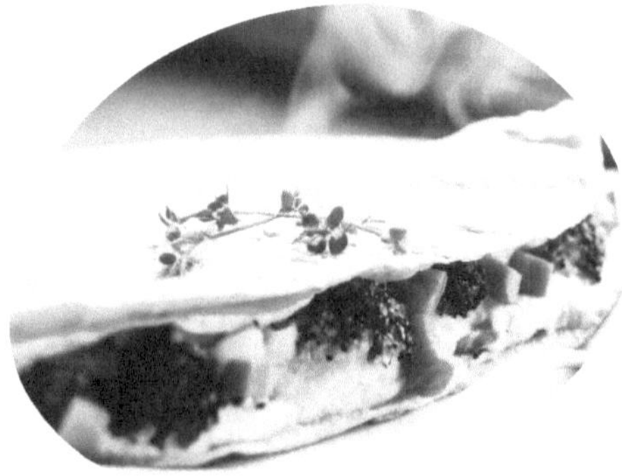

A colorful, soft omelet loaded with vegetables and light cheese.

Nutrition: 185 kcal, 16g protein, 9g fat, 8g carbs, 210mg sodium

INGREDIENTS

- 4 tbsp chopped broccoli
- 2 tbsp chopped onion
- 2 tbsp finely chopped carrot
- 4 egg whites
- 1 whole egg
- 1 oz light cheese
- Cooking spray

INSTRUCTIONS

- Heat a non-stick pan and spray lightly.
- Sauté broccoli, onion, and carrot until tender.
- Whisk eggs and season lightly.
- Pour eggs over vegetables and cook for three minutes.
- Add cheese, fold in half, and cook one more minute.
- Serve warm.

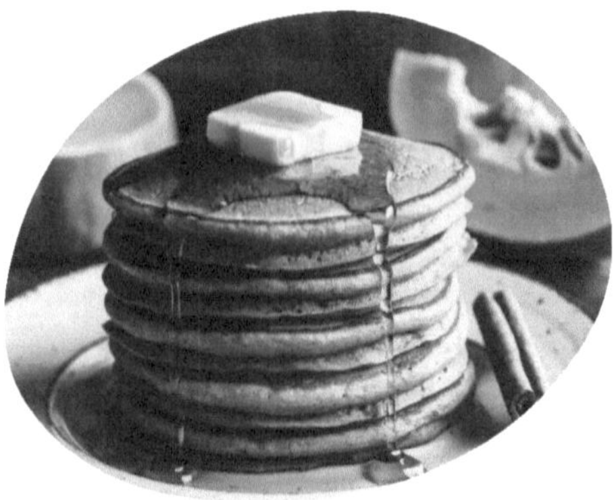

18. PUMPKIN MIX PANCAKES

Soft, aromatic pancakes filled with fiber and warm spices.

Nutrition: 200 kcal, 6g protein, 5g fat, 33g carbs, 190mg sodium

INGREDIENTS

- 1 egg
- ½ cup canned pumpkin
- 1¾ cups low-fat milk
- 2 tbsp vegetable oil
- 2 cups flour
- 2 tbsp brown sugar
- 1 tbsp baking powder
- 1 tsp pumpkin spice
- 1 tsp salt

INSTRUCTIONS

- Whisk egg, pumpkin, milk, and oil together.
- Add flour, sugar, baking powder, spice, and salt.
- Mix until just combined.
- Pour batter onto a greased skillet and cook until golden on both sides.
- Serve warm with fruit slices.

19. CHEESE MINI EGG AND BROCCOLI OMELET

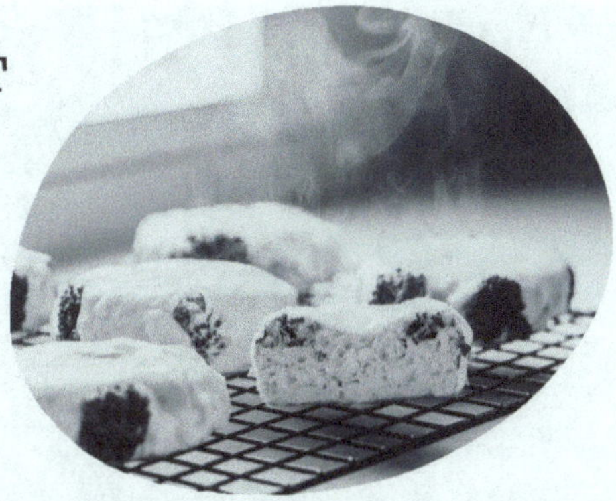

Mini baked omelets ideal for portion control and easy chewing.

Nutrition: 170 kcal, 15g protein, 9g fat, 4g carbs, 185mg sodium

INGREDIENTS

- 4 cups broccoli florets
- 4 whole eggs
- 1 cup egg whites
- 1/4 cup reduced-fat cheddar
- 1/4 cup grated parmesan
- 1 tbsp olive oil
- Salt and pepper to taste

INSTRUCTIONS

- Preheat oven to 350°F.
- Steam broccoli until soft, then chop finely.
- Mix with oil, salt, and pepper.
- Whisk eggs, whites, and cheese together.
- Spoon broccoli into muffin tins and pour egg mix over.
- Bake 20 minutes until firm.

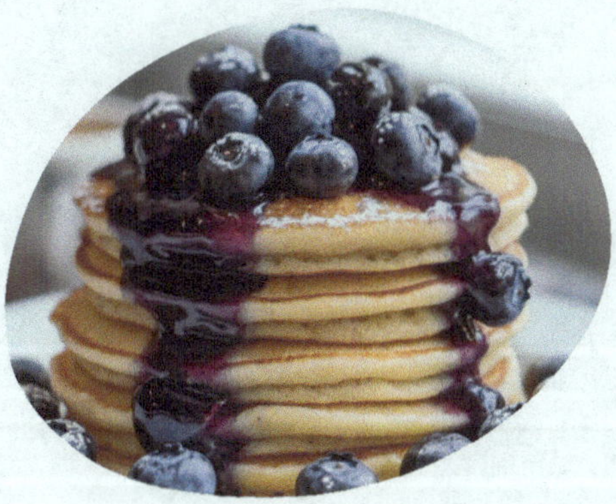

20. BLUEBERRY DOUBLE PANCAKES

Fluffy, antioxidant-rich pancakes with a natural blueberry topping.

Nutrition: 190 kcal, 7g protein, 6g fat, 29g carbs, 160mg sodium

INGREDIENTS

- 1 cup whole wheat flour
- 1 egg
- 1 cup low-fat yogurt
- 2 tbsp canola oil
- 1 tsp baking powder
- 1/2 tsp baking soda
- 1/4 tsp salt
- 1 cup fresh blueberries

INSTRUCTIONS

- Method:
- Whisk yogurt, egg, and oil in a bowl.
- Add flour, baking powder, soda, and salt.
- Mix until smooth.
- Stir in half the blueberries.
- Cook pancakes on a lightly greased pan until golden.
- Top with remaining blueberries before serving.

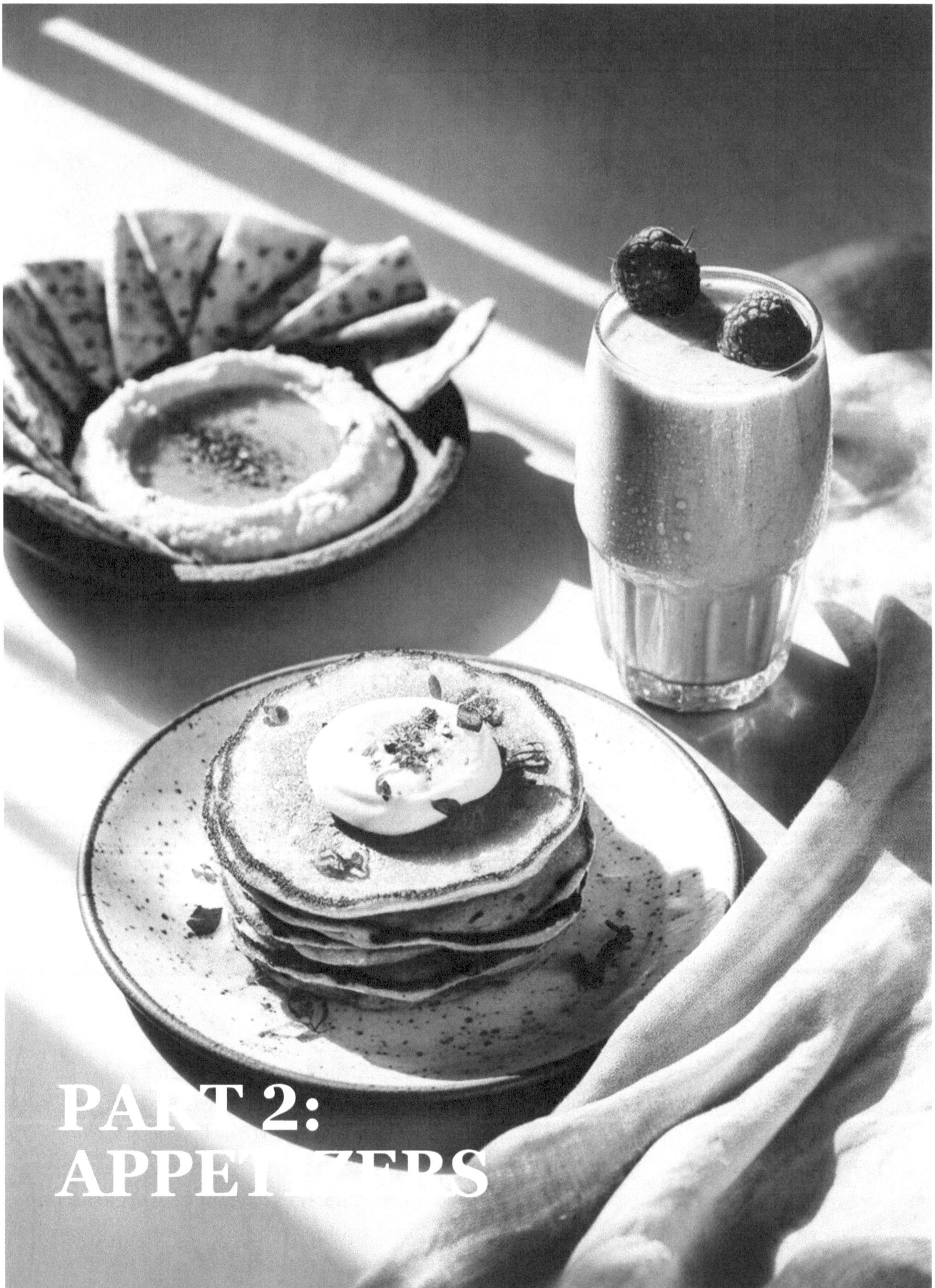

PART 2: APPETIZERS

1. FIESTA SURPRISE ROLL

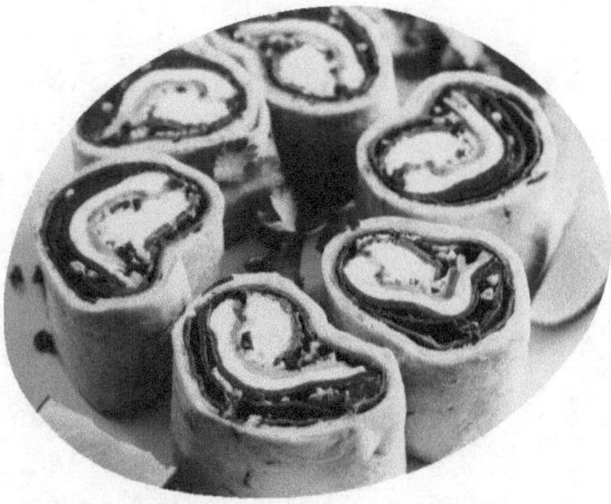

Colorful, flavorful, and packed with fiber and heart-healthy peppers.

Nutrition: 125 kcal, 5g protein, 4g fat, 15g carbs, 140mg sodium

INGREDIENTS

- 2 poblano peppers
- 2 red sweet peppers
- ½ cup fat-free cream cheese
- 1 tbsp chopped cilantro
- 2 tsp lime juice
- 1/8 tsp ground red pepper
- 2 cloves garlic, minced
- 4 whole wheat tortillas

INSTRUCTIONS

- Preheat oven to 425°F.
- Roast peppers cut-side down for 25 minutes until blistered.
- Cool, peel, and slice thinly.
- Mix cream cheese, cilantro, lime juice, pepper, and garlic.
- Spread mixture on tortillas, layer with peppers, and roll tightly.
- Wrap and chill 6 hours before slicing.

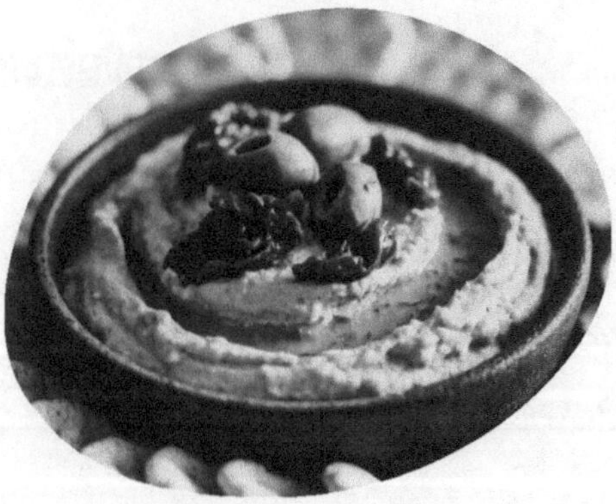

2. BEAN DIP AND OLIVE ATHENOS

Creamy and satisfying, this dip offers plant-based protein and flavor.

Nutrition: 150 kcal, 8g protein, 3g fat, 22g carbs, 160mg sodium

INGREDIENTS

- 3½ cups cooked garbanzo beans
- ⅔ cup fat-free sour cream
- 2 tsp minced garlic
- 4 tbsp balsamic vinegar
- ¼ cup chopped sun-dried tomatoes
- ¼ cup parsley
- 2 tbsp chopped Kalamata olives

INSTRUCTIONS

- Blend beans, sour cream, garlic, and vinegar until smooth.
- Stir in tomatoes, parsley, and olives.
- Chill 2 hours before serving.
- Enjoy with raw vegetables or whole-grain crackers.

3. STUFFED QUESADILLAS

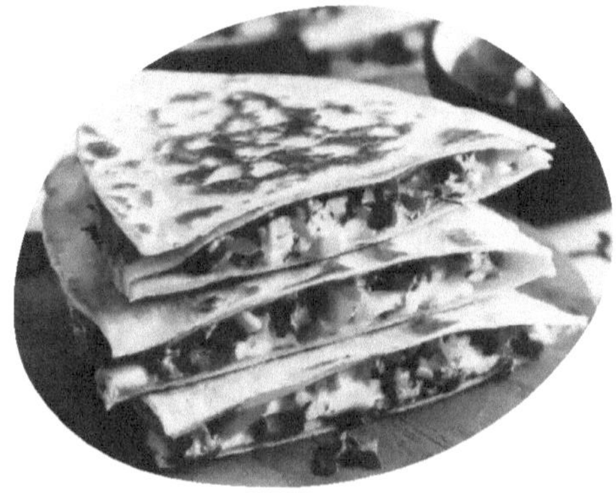

Crisp, cheesy, and packed with antioxidant-rich peppers.

Nutrition: 175 kcal, 6g protein, 7g fat, 20g carbs, 180mg sodium

INGREDIENTS

- 2 sweet peppers, thinly sliced
- 1 small red onion, sliced
- 2 tsp olive oil
- ½ tsp cumin
- ½ tsp chili powder
- 2 tbsp chopped parsley
- ⅓ cup reduced-fat cream cheese
- 5 small whole wheat tortillas

INSTRUCTIONS

- Sauté peppers and onions with olive oil and spices.
- Add parsley and cool slightly.
- Spread cream cheese on tortillas and top with pepper mixture.
- Fold and bake at 425°F for 6 minutes.
- Slice and serve warm with salsa.

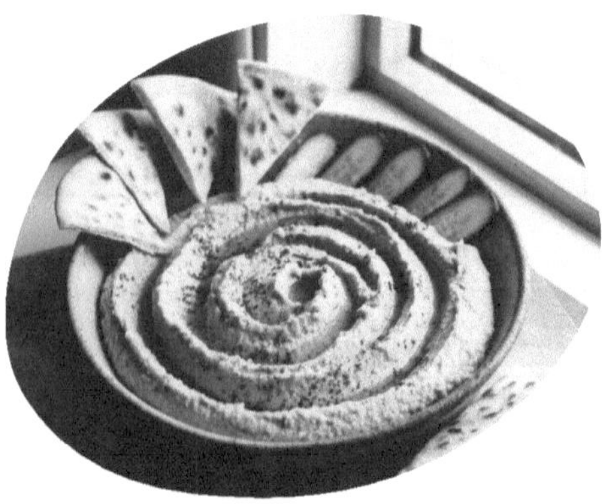

4. SESAME HUMMUS

Creamy, protein-rich, and excellent for dipping or spreading.

Nutrition: 140 kcal, 5g protein, 7g fat, 13g carbs, 135mg sodium

INGREDIENTS

- ¼ cup tahini
- 1 15-oz can garbanzo beans, rinsed
- 1/8 cup lemon juice
- ½ tsp garlic, minced
- ½ tsp salt
- 2 tbsp olive oil
- Pinch red chili flakes

INSTRUCTIONS

- Blend tahini, beans, lemon juice, garlic, and salt.
- Add olive oil and blend until smooth.
- Chill 1 hour before serving for best flavor.

5. ROASTED ALMONDS WITH ROSEMARY

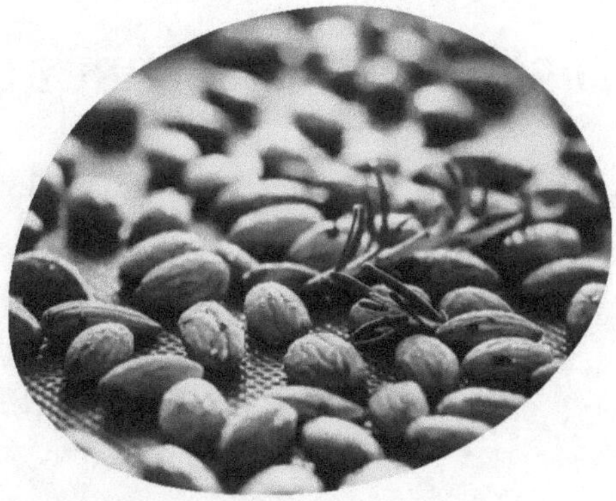

Crunchy, fragrant, and rich in healthy fats.

Nutrition: 190 kcal, 6g protein, 16g fat, 6g carbs, 120mg sodium

INGREDIENTS

- 1 tbsp chopped rosemary
- 1 tbsp olive oil
- 1 tsp chili powder
- ¾ tsp salt
- 2 cups almonds

INSTRUCTIONS

- Preheat oven to 325°F.
- Mix all ingredients in a bowl.
- Spread on baking sheet and roast 20 minutes.
- Cool before serving.

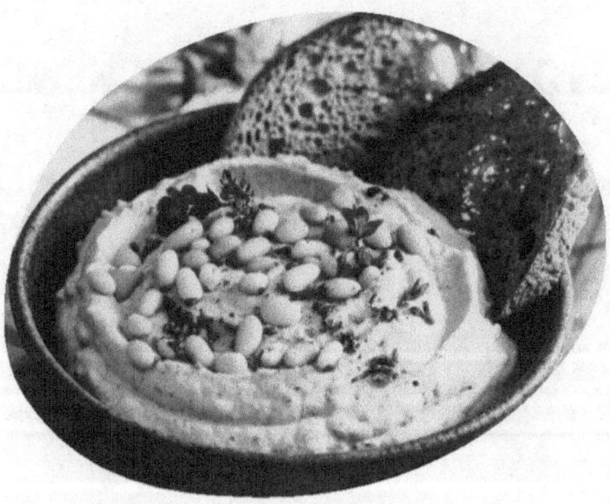

6. WHITE BEAN AND NUT DIP

A creamy, nutty spread that's low in sodium and high in protein.

Nutrition: 135 kcal, 7g protein, 5g fat, 16g carbs, 125mg sodium

INGREDIENTS

- 1 can white kidney beans, rinsed
- ¼ cup sour cream
- 3 tbsp toasted pine nuts
- ¼ cup bread crumbs
- 2 tbsp milk
- ¼ tsp garlic-herb seasoning
- ⅛ tsp cayenne pepper

INSTRUCTIONS

- Soak bread crumbs in milk.
- Blend beans, sour cream, nuts, seasoning, and pepper until smooth.
- Add soaked crumbs and blend again.
- Chill two hours before serving.

7. PEACH AND RASPBERRY LASSI

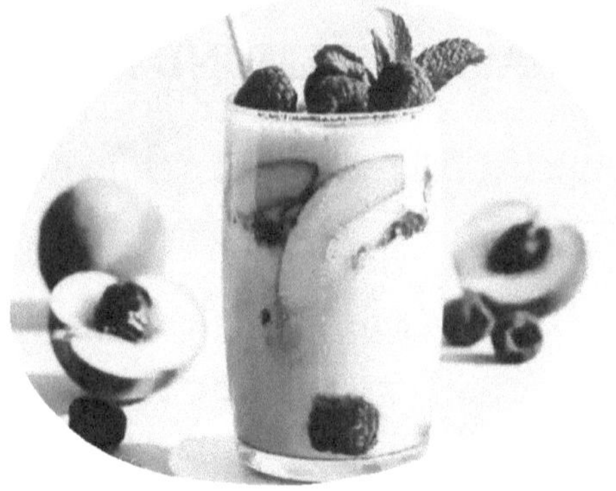

A fruity, refreshing drink packed with antioxidants.

Nutrition: 120 kcal, 4g protein, 2g fat, 21g carbs, 80mg sodium

INGREDIENTS

- 1 cup peaches
- ½ banana
- ½ cup raspberries
- 1 cup low-fat buttermilk
- 3 ice cubes

INSTRUCTIONS

- Combine all ingredients in a blender.
- Blend until smooth and creamy.
- Serve immediately chilled.

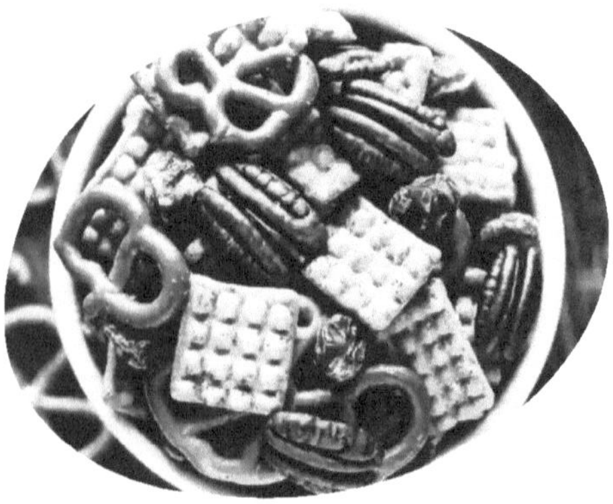

8. WAFERS AND CINNAMON SNACK MIX

A crunchy, sweet, and lightly spiced snack.

Nutrition: 180 kcal, 3g protein, 7g fat, 26g carbs, 150mg sodium

INGREDIENTS

- 3 cups whole-grain wafers
- 1 cup pecans
- 1 cup pretzel sticks
- 3 tbsp melted butter
- 2 tbsp sugar
- 1 tsp cinnamon
- ¼ tsp salt
- ½ cup yogurt-covered raisins

INSTRUCTIONS

- Preheat oven to 375°F.
- Toss wafers, nuts, and pretzels.
- Mix butter, cinnamon, sugar, and salt.
- Combine and bake for 10 minutes.
- Cool and mix in raisins.

9. PUMPKIN VANILLA SMOOTHIE

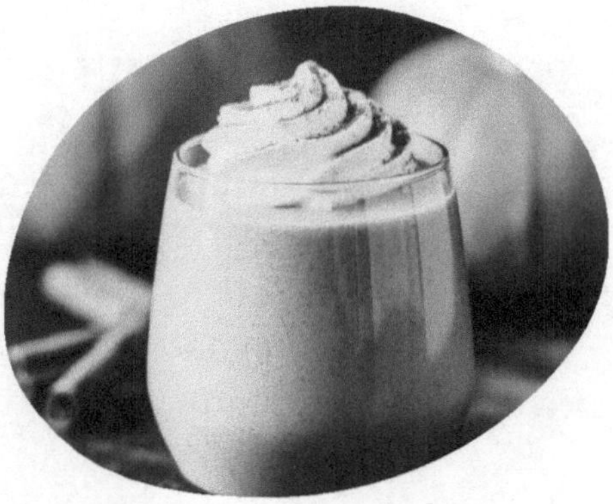

Creamy and lightly spiced, perfect for heart-healthy energy.

*Nutrition: 160 kcal, 7g protein, \
3g fat, 28g carbs, 110mg sodium*

INGREDIENTS

- 1 cup milk
- ¾ cup vanilla yogurt
- ½ cup canned pumpkin
- 1 banana
- 1 tbsp maple syrup
- ½ tsp pumpkin spice
- Ice cubes

INSTRUCTIONS

- Blend milk, yogurt, pumpkin, banana, syrup, and spice.
- Add ice cubes for desired consistency.
- Blend until smooth and serve.

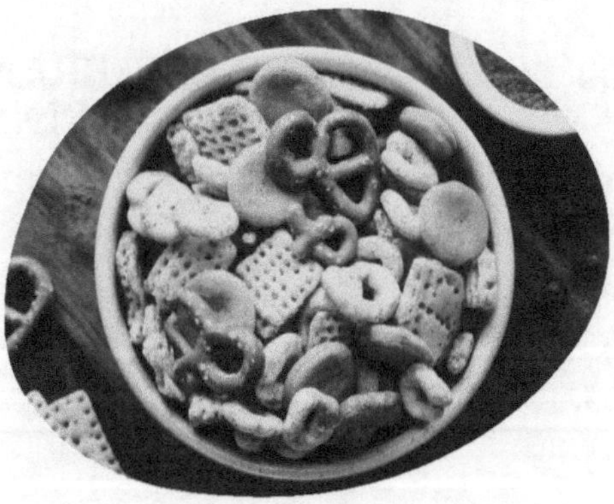

10. SNACK CURRY MIX

Crispy, flavorful, and easy to make with minimal salt.

*Nutrition: 125 kcal, 3g protein,
4g fat, 19g carbs, 140mg sodium*

INGREDIENTS

- 3 rice cakes, broken
- 1 cup corn cereal
- ¾ cup pretzel sticks
- 1 tbsp melted margarine
- 1 tsp Worcestershire sauce
- ½ tsp curry powder

INSTRUCTIONS

- Preheat oven to 300°F.
- Mix cereal, rice cakes, and pretzels.
- Blend margarine with sauce and curry powder.
- Pour over mixture and bake 20 minutes.
- Cool before serving.

11. POPCORN SNACK MIX

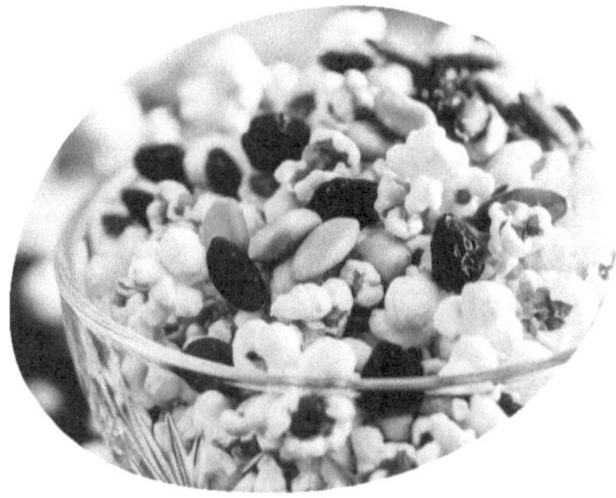

Light, crunchy, and full of fiber and healthy fats.

Nutrition: 160 kcal, 6g protein, 7g fat, 21g carbs, 125mg sodium

INGREDIENTS

- 10 cups air-popped popcorn
- 1 tbsp taco seasoning
- 1 cup peanuts
- 1/2 cup pumpkin seeds
- 1 cup golden raisins

INSTRUCTIONS

- Coat popcorn lightly with spray.
- Toss with taco seasoning.
- Add peanuts, seeds, and raisins.
- Mix well and serve immediately.

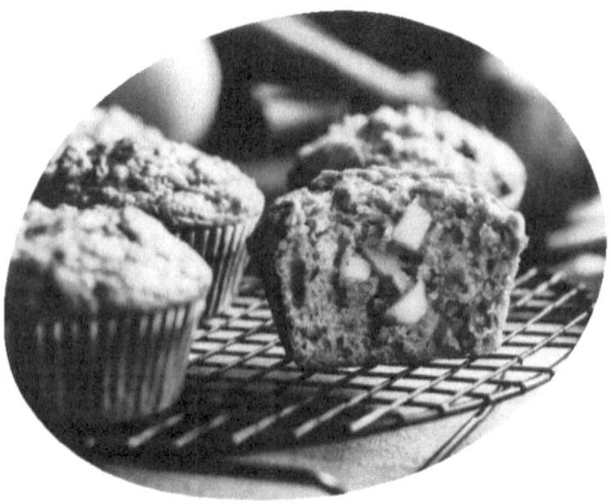

12. APPLE BUTTERMILK AND OAT BRAN MUFFINS

Soft, fiber-rich muffins with gentle sweetness and spice.

Nutrition: 160 kcal, 5g protein, 4g fat, 28g carbs, 120mg sodium

INGREDIENTS

- 3/4 cup all-purpose flour
- 3/4 cup whole wheat flour
- 1 cup buttermilk
- 1/2 cup oat bran
- 1/4 cup brown sugar
- 2 tbsp oil
- 1 egg
- 1 1/2 cups chopped apples
- 1 1/2 tsp cinnamon
- 1 tsp baking powder

INSTRUCTIONS

- Preheat oven to 400°F.
- Mix dry ingredients in one bowl.
- Combine wet ingredients and apples in another.
- Blend together and fill muffin cups.
- Bake 20 minutes until golden

13. SWEET WHEAT MUFFINS

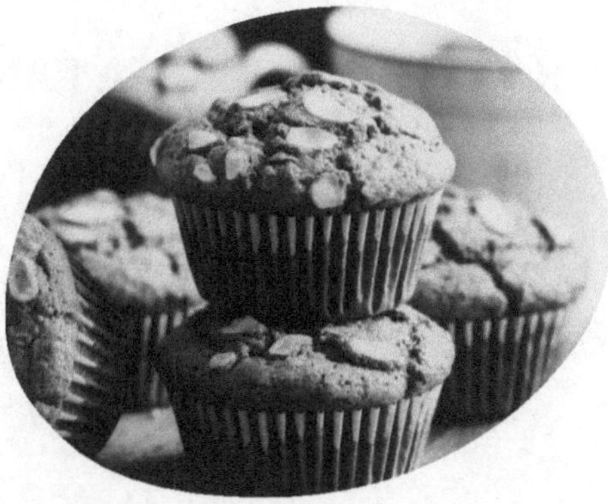

Whole-grain muffins that support healthy aging and digestion.

Nutrition: 155 kcal, 4g protein, 3g fat, 27g carbs, 130mg sodium

INGREDIENTS

- 2 cups whole wheat flour
- 1/2 cup sugar
- 3 1/2 tsp baking powder
- 2 egg whites
- 3 tbsp canola oil
- 1 1/3 cups skim milk with 1 tbsp vinegar

INSTRUCTIONS

- Preheat oven to 350°F.
- Mix flour, sugar, and baking powder.
- Whisk milk, oil, and egg whites.
- Combine wet and dry ingredients.
- Spoon into muffin cups and bake 25 minutes.

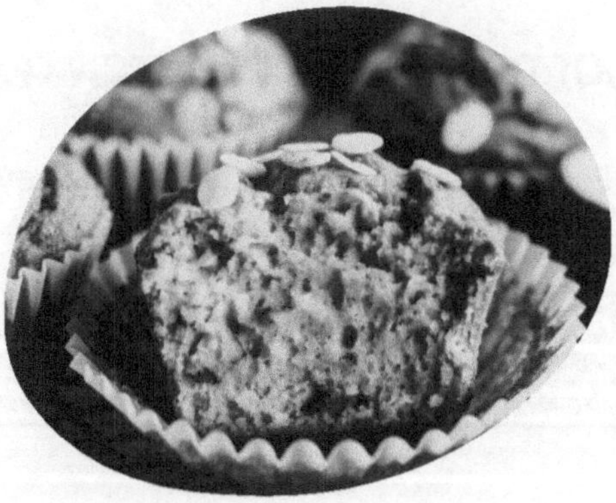

14. ZUCCHINI CINNAMON MUFFINS

Moist, fragrant muffins high in fiber and low in sugar.

Nutrition: 165 kcal, 4g protein, 4g fat, 28g carbs, 125mg sodium

INGREDIENTS

- 1 cup all-purpose flour
- 1 cup whole wheat flour
- 1/2 tsp cinnamon
- 1/4 tsp nutmeg
- 1 1/2 tsp baking powder
- 1/2 tsp baking soda
- 1 egg
- 3/4 cup low-fat milk
- 1 cup shredded zucchini
- 2 tbsp canola oil

INSTRUCTIONS

- Preheat oven to 400°F.
- Mix dry ingredients.
- Whisk wet ingredients separately.
- Combine both and fold in zucchini.
- Bake 25 minutes until light brown.

15. ROASTED CHICKPEA PANCAKES

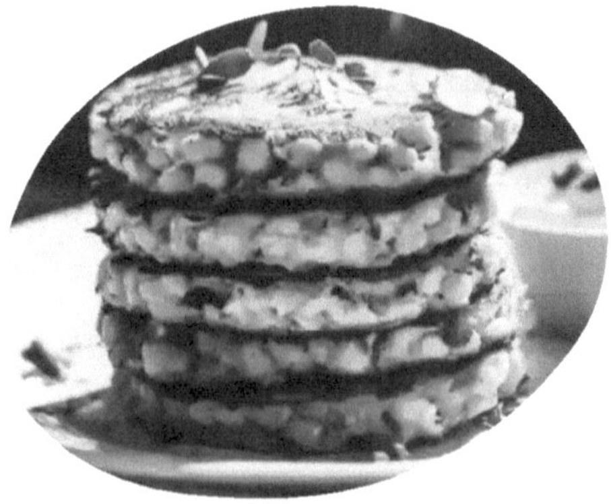

Savory, protein-rich, and packed with fiber and flavor.

Nutrition: 170 kcal, 9g protein, 6g fat, 20g carbs, 140mg sodium

INGREDIENTS

- 1 cup canned chickpeas, drained
- ½ cup flour
- ½ tsp cumin
- 2 eggs
- ¼ cup chickpea liquid
- 2 tbsp tahini
- Juice of 1 lemon

INSTRUCTIONS

- Blend chickpeas, tahini, lemon juice, and eggs until smooth.
- Mix in flour and cumin.
- Cook pancakes on a lightly oiled skillet, 2 minutes per side.
- Serve warm with yogurt dip.

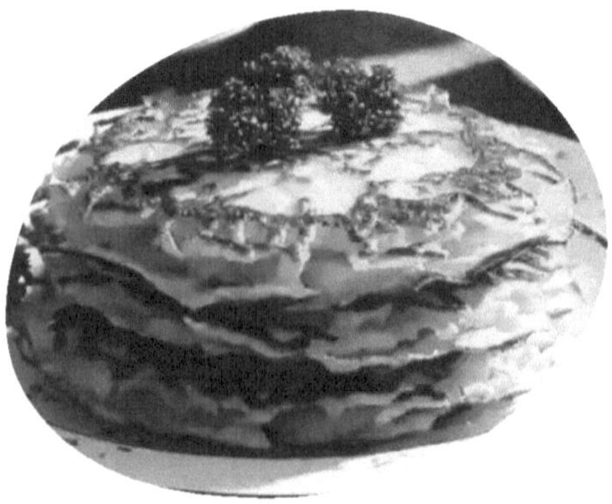

16. GOLDEN POTATO PANCAKES

Crisp outside, tender inside, and easy to chew.

Nutrition: 185 kcal, 5g protein, 6g fat, 27g carbs, 160mg sodium

INGREDIENTS

- 6 boiled potatoes, mashed
- 2 eggs
- ¼ cup whole wheat bread crumbs
- 1 tbsp parsley
- ¼ cup flour
- 2 tbsp canola oil

INSTRUCTIONS

- Mix potatoes, eggs, parsley, and bread crumbs.
- Form small patties and coat with flour.
- Pan-fry in oil 3 minutes per side until golden.
- Serve warm.

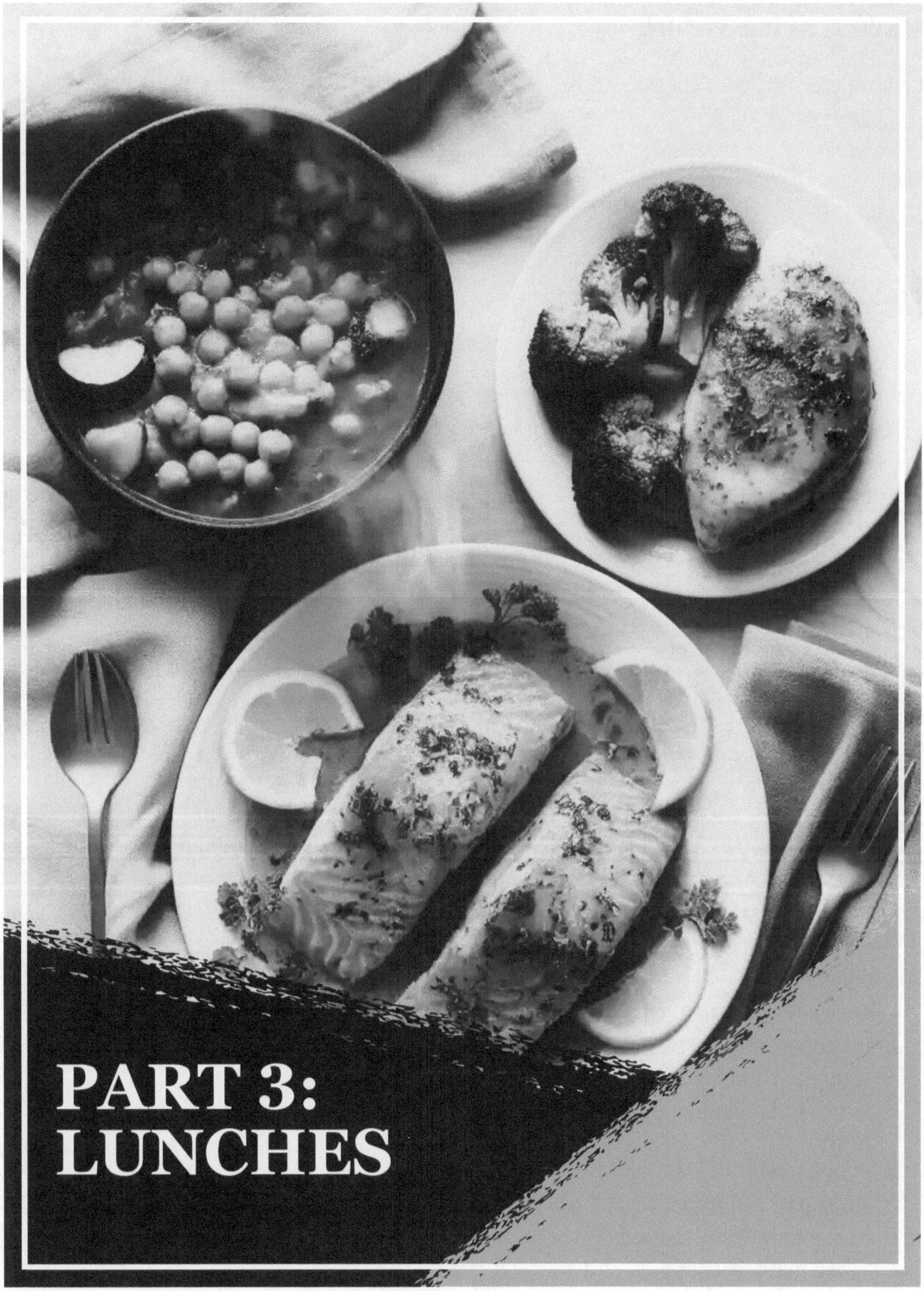

PART 3: LUNCHES

1. SWISS APPLE PANINI

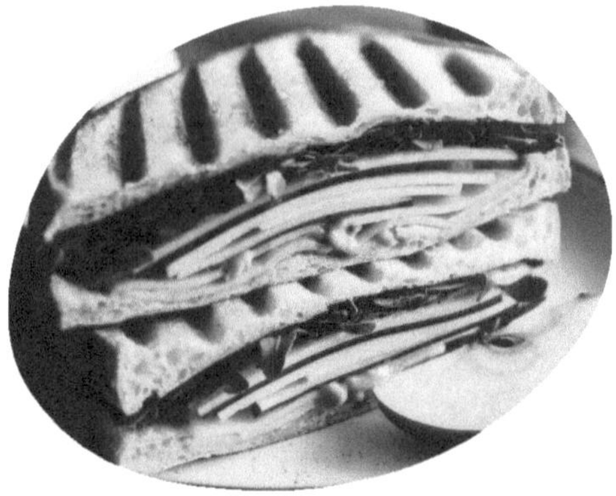

Crisp apple and Swiss cheese panini.

Nutrition: 280 kcal, 16g protein, 7g fat, 36g carbs, 310mg sodium

INGREDIENTS

- 8 slices whole-grain bread
- 1/4 cup non-fat honey mustard
- 2 crisp apples, thinly sliced
- 6 oz low-fat Swiss cheese, thinly sliced
- 1 cup arugula leaves
- Cooking spray

INSTRUCTIONS

- Preheat a Panini press or skillet.
- Spread honey mustard evenly on each bread slice.
- Layer cheese, apple, and arugula on 4 slices and top with remaining bread.
- Lightly coat your press with cooking spray.
- Grill sandwiches for 3 to 5 minutes until cheese melts and bread turns golden.
- Cool slightly before serving.

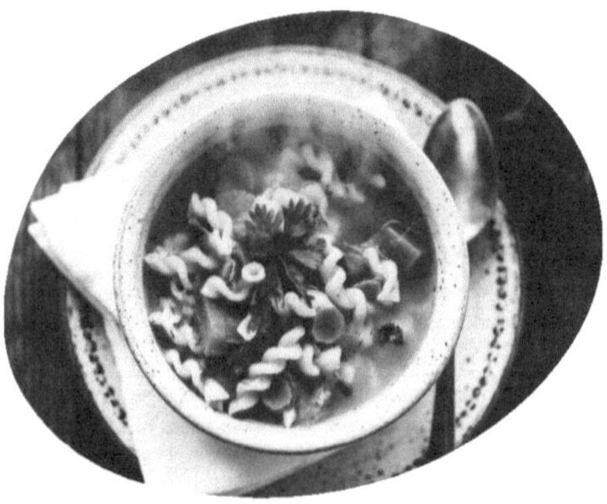

2. VEGETARIAN PASTA SOUP

Light soup with vegetables and pasta.

Nutrition: 230 kcal, 9g protein, 6g fat, 34g carbs, 280mg sodium

INGREDIENTS

- 2 tsp olive oil
- 6 garlic cloves, minced
- 1½ cups shredded carrot
- 1 cup each chopped onion and celery
- 1 box (32 oz) low-sodium chicken broth
- 4 cups water
- 1½ cups ditalini pasta
- 1/4 cup Parmesan, shaved
- 2 tbsp parsley, chopped

INSTRUCTIONS

- Heat olive oil in a Dutch oven over medium heat.
- Add garlic, carrot, onion, and celery; sauté 5 to 7 minutes.
- Add broth and water; bring to a boil.
- Add pasta and cook 7 to 8 minutes until tender.
- Top each serving with Parmesan and parsley.

3. GRILLED VEGGIE TOAST CALIFORNIAN-STYLE

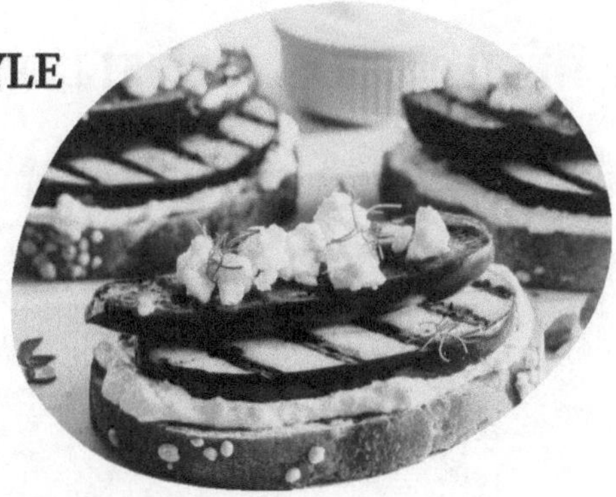

Focaccia topped with grilled vegetables.

Nutrition: 310 kcal, 11g protein, 17g fat, 27g carbs, 340mg sodium

INGREDIENTS

- 3 tbsp light mayonnaise
- 3 cloves garlic, minced
- 1 tbsp lemon juice
- 1/8 cup olive oil
- 1 cup red bell pepper, sliced
- 1 small zucchini, sliced
- 1 yellow squash, sliced
- 2 slices whole wheat focaccia
- ½ cup crumbled feta cheese

INSTRUCTIONS

- Mix mayonnaise, lemon juice, and garlic; refrigerate.
- Brush vegetables with olive oil and grill 3 minutes per side until tender.
- Spread garlic mayo on focaccia slices and top with feta.
- Grill bread for 3 minutes until cheese softens.
- Layer vegetables and serve open-faced.

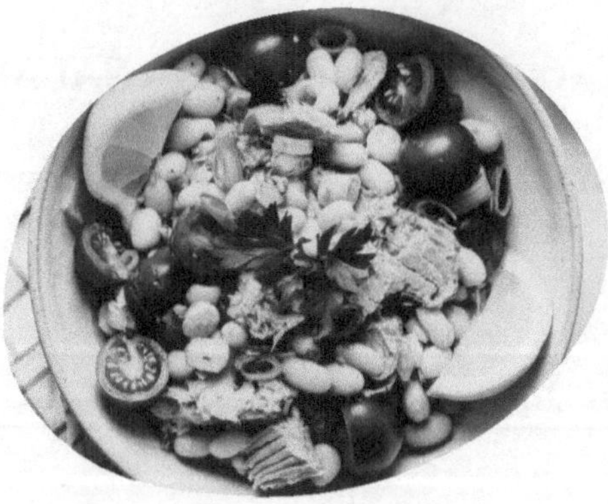

4. TUNA SALAD TUSCAN-STYLE

Fresh tuna and white bean salad.

Nutrition: 240 kcal, 23g protein, 9g fat, 17g carbs, 290mg sodium

INGREDIENTS

- 2 cans (6 oz each) light tuna, drained
- 1 can (15 oz) small white beans, rinsed
- 10 cherry tomatoes, quartered
- 4 scallions, sliced
- 2 tbsp olive oil
- 2 tbsp lemon juice
- ¼ tsp salt
- Black pepper

INSTRUCTIONS

- Combine tuna, beans, tomatoes, and scallions.
- Drizzle with olive oil and lemon juice, and season with salt and pepper.
- Toss gently and refrigerate before serving.

5. DELIGHTFUL TORTELLINI SALAD

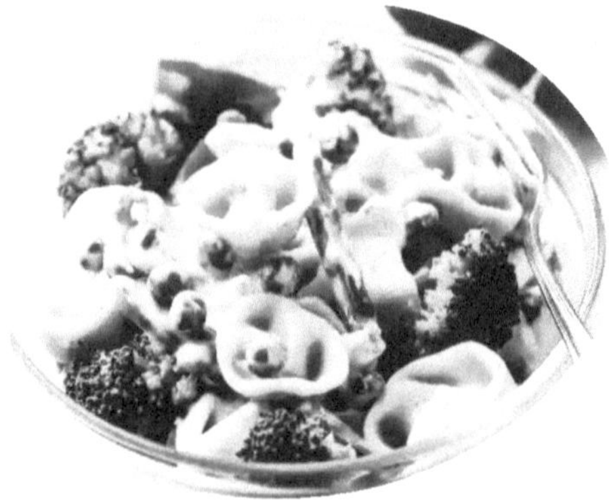

Creamy tortellini with broccoli and carrots.

Nutrition: 270 kcal, 12g protein, 9g fat, 33g carbs, 360mg sodium

INGREDIENTS

- 1 package (9 oz) light cheese tortellini
- 3 cups broccoli florets
- 1 cup sliced carrots
- 1/4 cup green onions
- 1/2 cup low-fat ranch dressing
- 1 large tomato, chopped
- 1 cup pea pods, halved

INSTRUCTIONS

- Cook pasta per package directions; add carrots and broccoli for last 3 minutes.
- Drain and rinse with cold water.
- Toss pasta and onions with ranch dressing.
- Chill 2 hours, then add tomato and pea pods before serving.

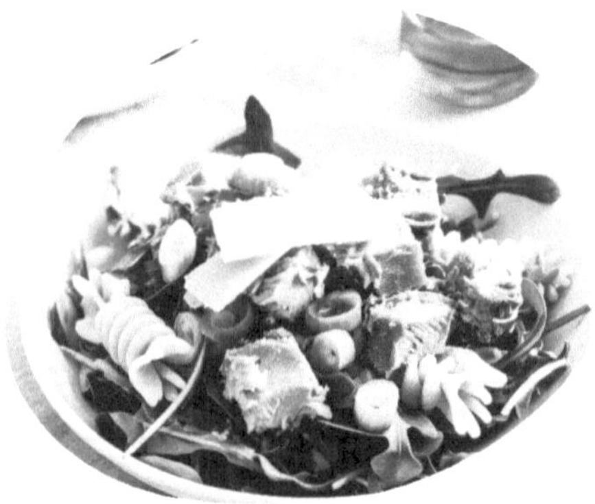

6. HEALTHY TUNA SALAD

Simple tuna and arugula pasta bowl.

Nutrition: 220 kcal, 20g protein, 8g fat, 18g carbs, 260mg sodium

INGREDIENTS

- 5 oz can light tuna, drained
- 1 tbsp olive oil
- 1 tbsp red wine vinegar
- 1/4 cup chopped green onions
- 2 cups arugula
- 1 cup cooked pasta
- 1 tbsp Parmesan cheese
- Black pepper

INSTRUCTIONS

- Combine tuna, oil, vinegar, arugula, onion, and pasta.
- Divide between two plates and garnish with Parmesan and pepper.

7. AVOCADO, STRAWBERRY & MELON SALAD

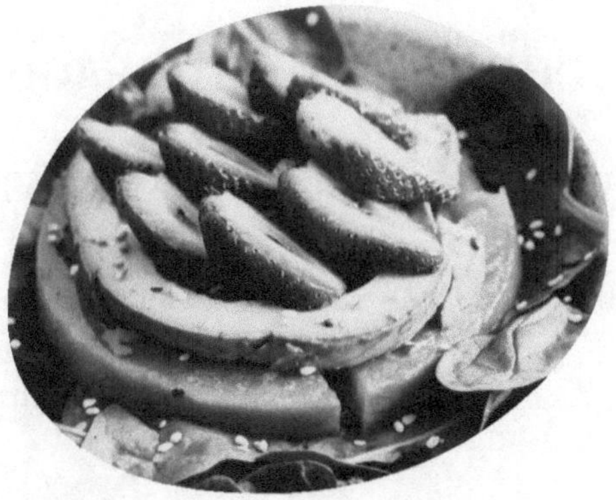

Fruity spinach salad with avocado slices.

Nutrition: 190 kcal, 4g protein, 8g fat, 28g carbs, 120mg sodium

INGREDIENTS

- 1/4 cup honey
- 2 tbsp sherry vinegar
- 2 tbsp chopped mint
- Black pepper and salt to taste
- 4 cups baby spinach
- 1 small avocado, sliced
- 16 slices cantaloupe
- 1 1/2 cups strawberries, sliced
- 2 tsp toasted sesame seeds

INSTRUCTIONS

- Whisk honey, vinegar, mint, pepper, and salt.
- Divide spinach among plates, layer avocado, cantaloupe, and strawberries.
- Drizzle dressing and sprinkle sesame seeds before serving.

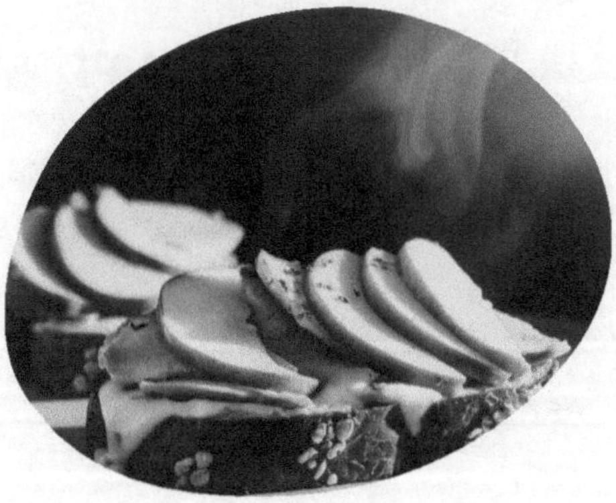

8. CHEESY PEAR & TURKEY SANDWICH

Melted turkey, pear, and mozzarella toast.

Nutrition: 260 kcal, 20g protein, 6g fat, 29g carbs, 290mg sodium

INGREDIENTS

- 2 slices whole wheat bread
- 2 tsp Dijon mustard
- 2 slices (1 oz each) low-sodium turkey
- 1 pear, thinly sliced
- 1/4 cup shredded mozzarella
- Black pepper

INSTRUCTIONS

- Spread mustard on bread, top each slice with turkey and pear.
- Sprinkle cheese and pepper.
- Broil 2 to 3 minutes until cheese melts.
- Cut in half and serve open-faced.

9. CHUNKY TOMATO SPAGHETTI SQUASH

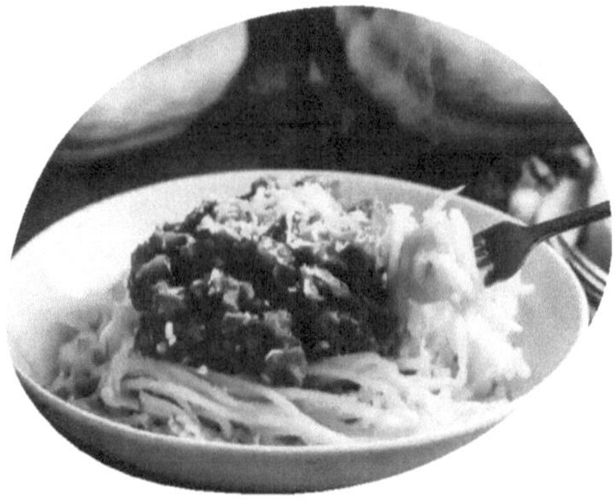

Tomato-beef sauce over tender squash.

Nutrition: 290 kcal, 23g protein, 9g fat, 28g carbs, 320mg sodium

INGREDIENTS

- 1 lb lean ground beef
- ½ cup chopped onion
- ½ cup green pepper
- 2 cloves garlic, minced
- 1 can (14 oz) diced tomatoes
- 1 can (8 oz) tomato sauce
- Italian seasoning and black pepper
- 1 cooked spaghetti squash
- ¼ cup Parmesan cheese

INSTRUCTIONS

- Cook beef, onion, garlic, and pepper until browned; drain.
- Add tomatoes, sauce, paste, and seasoning; simmer 15 minutes.
- Serve over squash and top with Parmesan.

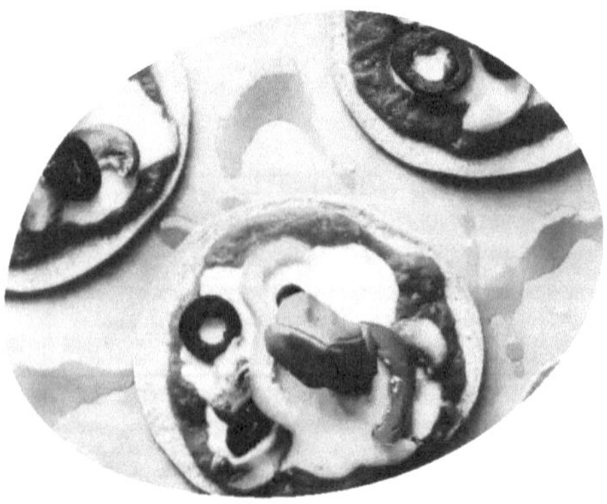

10. PITA PIZZA

Whole wheat pita topped with veggies.

Nutrition: 230 kcal, 13g protein, 8g fat, 26g carbs, 270mg sodium

INGREDIENTS

- 2 whole wheat pitas
- ¼ cup tomato sauce
- ½ cup mozzarella
- Vegetables of choice (bell pepper, onion, olives, mushrooms)

INSTRUCTIONS

- Preheat oven to 350°F.
- Spread sauce and cheese inside pita halves with toppings.
- Wrap in foil and bake for 7 to 10 minutes.

11. MUSHROOM, TOFU & SPINACH SOBA MIX

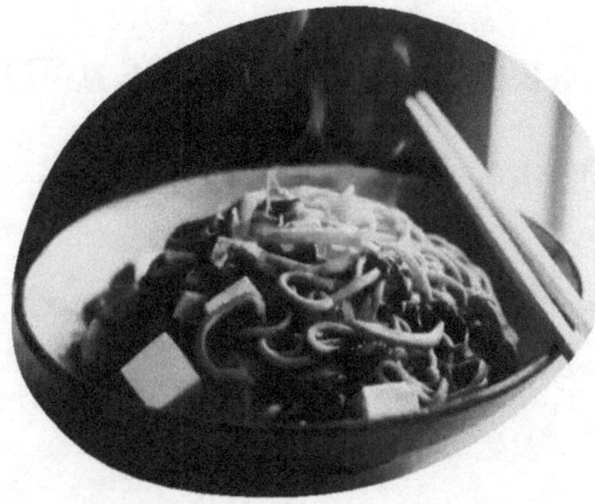

Soba noodles with tofu and mushrooms.

Nutrition: 330 kcal, 20g protein, 9g fat, 41g carbs, 310mg sodium

INGREDIENTS

- 2 tbsp canola oil
- 1 shallot, minced
- 1 carrot, diced
- 2 cloves garlic, minced
- 1½ tbsp fresh ginger
- 8 oz mushrooms, sliced
- 1 cup edamame
- 1½ cups vegetable broth
- 2 tbsp soy sauce (low sodium)
- 1 tsp lemon zest
- 4 oz spinach, chopped
- 4 oz firm tofu, diced
- 6 oz soba noodles

INSTRUCTIONS

- Sauté shallot, carrot, garlic, and ginger in oil.
- Add mushrooms and cook covered until tender.
- Add edamame, broth, lemon zest, and soy sauce.
- Stir in spinach and tofu; heat through.
- Boil soba noodles separately, drain, and toss into pan.

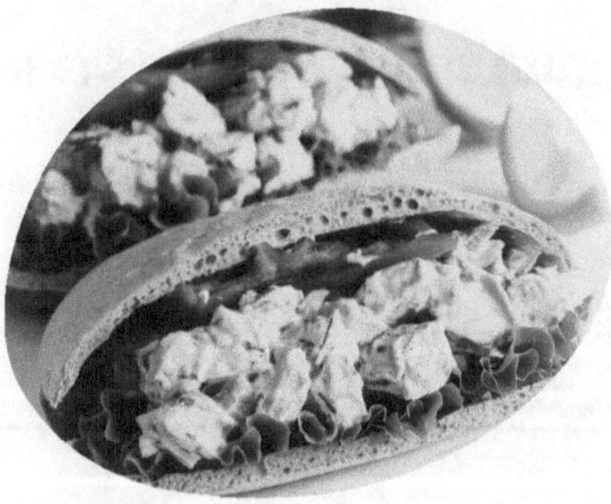

12. SALMON SALAD IN A PITA

Creamy salmon wrap with crisp lettuce.

Nutrition: 210 kcal, 20g protein, 5g fat, 18g carbs, 240mg sodium

INGREDIENTS

- ¾ cup canned salmon
- 3 tbsp fat-free yogurt
- 1 tbsp lemon juice
- 2 tbsp red bell pepper, minced
- 1 tbsp red onion, minced
- 1 tsp chopped capers
- Pinch dill
- Black pepper
- 3 lettuce leaves
- 3 small whole wheat pitas

INSTRUCTIONS

- Mix salmon, yogurt, lemon juice, pepper, onion, capers, and dill.
- Place lettuce and ⅓ cup filling in each pita pocket.

13. SKILLET POTATOES AND SAUSAGE

Golden potatoes with lean turkey sausage.

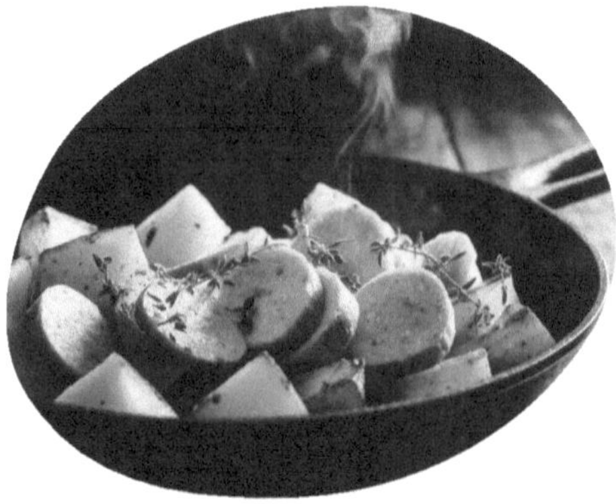

Nutrition: 310 kcal, 14g protein, 14g fat, 34g carbs, 380mg sodium

INGREDIENTS

- 1/2 lb cooked smoked low-sodium turkey sausage
- 3 tbsp olive oil
- 1 3/4 lbs red potatoes, unpeeled
- 2 medium onions
- 1 tsp dried thyme
- 1 1/2 tsp cumin seed, crushed
- 1/4 tsp salt
- 1/4 tsp black pepper

INSTRUCTIONS

- Cut potatoes into 1/2-inch cubes and slice onions. Heat oil in a large skillet and add potatoes and onions.
- Cook uncovered over medium-high heat for 12 minutes until nearly tender.
- Add sliced sausage and cook until potatoes are golden.
- Stir in thyme, cumin, salt, and pepper.
- Cook 1 more minute before serving

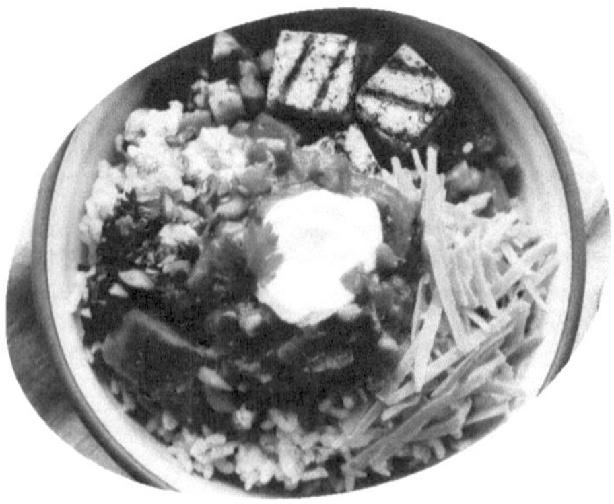

14. RICE BOWL, SOUTHWEST-STYLE

Colorful rice bowl with salsa topping.

Nutrition: 295 kcal, 20g protein, 8g fat, 35g carbs, 340mg sodium

INGREDIENTS

- 1 tsp vegetable oil
- 1 cup chopped mixed vegetables
- 1 cup cooked lean meat or tofu
- 1 cup cooked brown rice
- 4 tbsp salsa
- 2 tbsp shredded cheese
- 2 tbsp low-fat sour cream

INSTRUCTIONS

- Heat oil in skillet over medium heat.
- Add vegetables and cook 3–5 minutes until tender-crisp.
- Add meat and rice, stir until heated through.
- Divide between bowls and top with salsa, cheese, and sour cream.

15. SIRLOIN POTAGE

Hearty beef soup with garden vegetables.

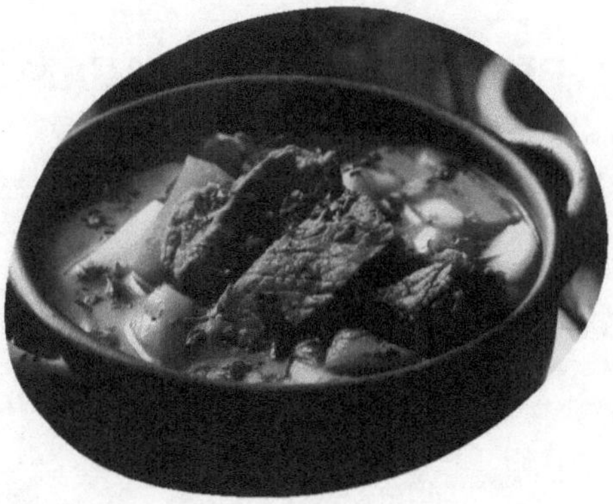

Nutrition: 280 kcal, 22g protein, 11g fat, 23g carbs, 370mg sodium

INGREDIENTS

- 1 tbsp oil
- 1 small onion, diced
- 1 lb lean ground sirloin
- 1/3 cup flour
- 1 carton (32 oz) beef broth
- 1 bag (1 lb) frozen soup vegetables
- 2 tbsp Worcestershire sauce

INSTRUCTIONS

- Heat oil and sauté onion until soft.
- Add ground beef and cook until browned.
- Shake flour with water and add to beef with broth.
- Stir and bring to a boil.
- Add vegetables and simmer 10 minutes.
- Finish with Worcestershire sauce.

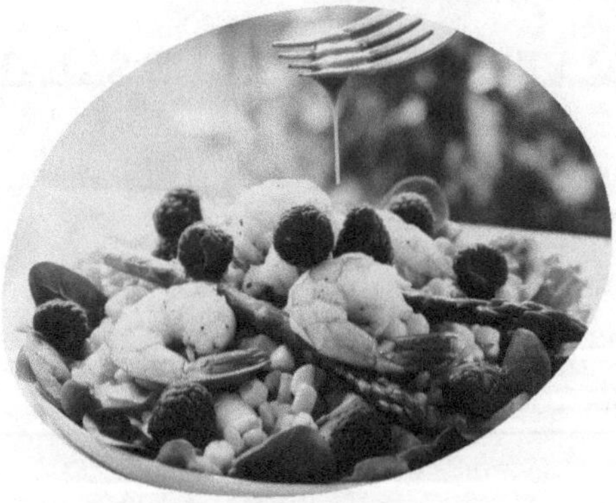

16. SHRIMP, CORN & RASPBERRY SALAD

Sweet berries with shrimp and greens.

Nutrition: 260 kcal, 21g protein, 10g fat, 20g carbs, 240mg sodium

INGREDIENTS

- 12 oz asparagus spears
- 1 cup baby corn
- 12 lettuce leaves
- 12 spinach leaves
- 12 oz shrimp, cooked
- 2 1/2 cups raspberries or strawberries
- 1/4 cup walnut oil
- 1/4 cup raspberry vinegar
- 1 tbsp chopped parsley
- 2 tsp honey

INSTRUCTIONS

- Cook asparagus and corn until crisp-tender, then cool.
- Arrange greens on plates and top with shrimp, corn, and berries.
- Whisk oil, vinegar, parsley, and honey for dressing.
- Drizzle dressing and serve chilled.

17. BLACK BEAN & GUACAMOLE CAKE

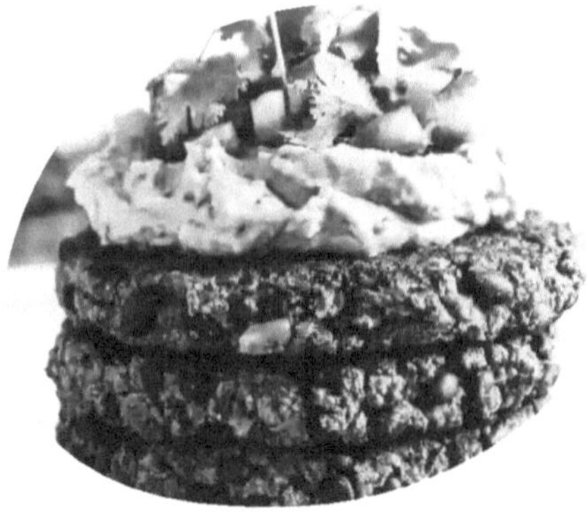

Smoky bean patties with avocado dip.

Nutrition: 240 kcal, 10g protein, 9g fat, 29g carbs, 260mg sodium

INGREDIENTS

- 2 slices whole wheat bread, torn
- 3 tbsp chopped cilantro
- 2 cloves garlic
- 1 can (15 oz) black beans, rinsed
- 1 chipotle pepper in adobo
- 1 tsp cumin
- 1 egg
- ½ avocado, mashed
- 1 tbsp lime juice
- 1 small tomato, diced

INSTRUCTIONS

- Blend bread into crumbs; transfer to bowl.
- Puree beans, cilantro, garlic, chipotle, and cumin.
- Add egg and mix with crumbs to form patties.
- Grill patties 8 minutes until heated through.
- Mash avocado with lime juice and serve with tomato on top.

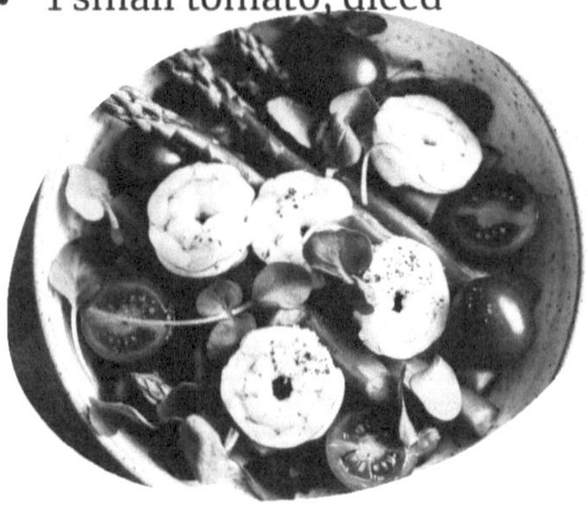

18. SHRIMP, TOMATO & ASPARAGUS SALAD

Shrimp salad with tomato and asparagus.

Nutrition: 220 kcal, 20g protein, 6g fat, 15g carbs, 250mg sodium

INGREDIENTS

- 12 oz asparagus spears
- 4 cups watercress
- 16 oz cooked shrimp
- 2 cups cherry tomatoes, halved
- ½ cup light raspberry vinaigrette
- Cracked black pepper

INSTRUCTIONS

- Steam asparagus for 3 minutes, then cool.
- Divide asparagus, shrimp, tomatoes, and watercress among plates.
- Drizzle vinaigrette and sprinkle pepper before serving.

19. CHEESY MUSHROOM & SPINACH WRAPS

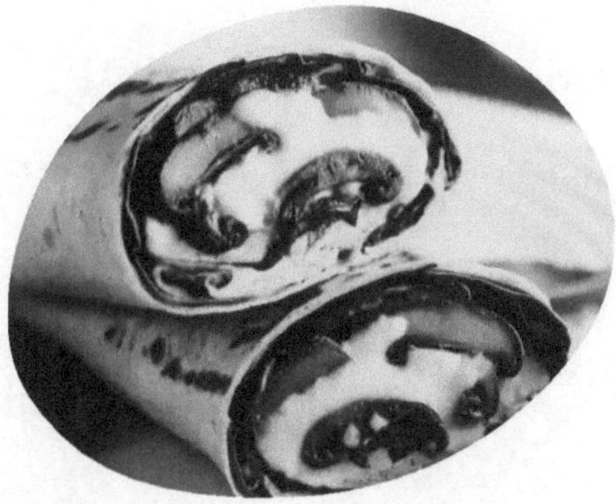

Warm wraps with spinach and cheese.

Nutrition: 265 kcal, 13g protein, 8g fat, 32g carbs, 280mg sodium

INGREDIENTS

- 1 tbsp olive oil
- 8 oz mushrooms, sliced
- 1 tsp minced garlic
- 2 whole wheat tortillas
- ½ lb spinach, steamed
- 1 tomato, diced
- ¼ cup shredded mozzarella

INSTRUCTIONS

- Heat olive oil, add garlic and mushrooms, and sauté until browned.
- Arrange spinach, mushrooms, tomato, and cheese on tortillas.
- Roll and bake at 350°F for 10 minutes.
- Cut into quarters and serve warm.

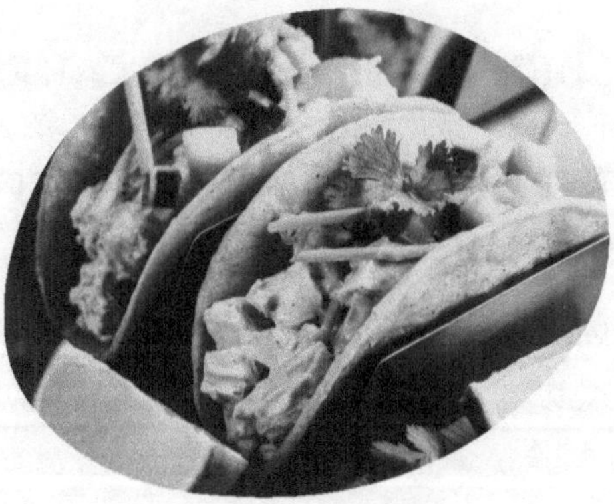

20. TACO CHICKEN SALAD

Zesty chicken salad in taco shells.

Nutrition: 180 kcal, 15g protein, 6g fat, 16g carbs, 260mg sodium

INGREDIENTS

- ⅓ cup cooked shredded chicken
- 2 tbsp chopped celery
- 1 tbsp light mayo
- 1 tbsp salsa
- 1 tbsp shredded cheddar
- 4 mini taco shells

INSTRUCTIONS

- Combine chicken, celery, mayo, salsa, and cheese.
- Spoon mixture into taco shells just before serving.

21. SUNSHINE IN A WRAP

Chicken wrap with oranges and celery.

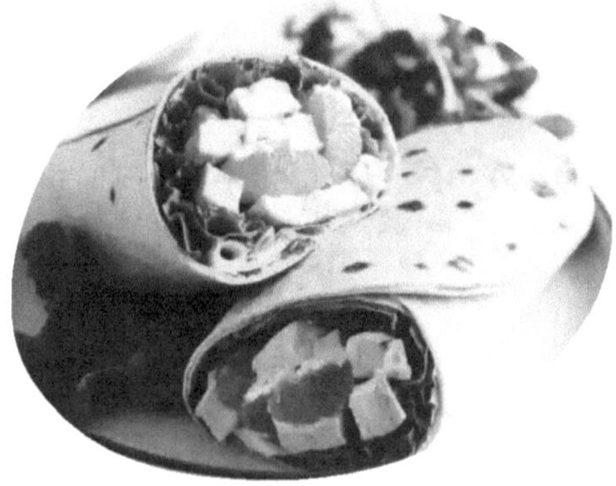

Nutrition: 275 kcal, 24g protein, 8g fat, 26g carbs, 290mg sodium

INGREDIENTS

- 8 oz cooked chicken breast
- 1/2 cup celery, diced
- 2/3 cup mandarin oranges, drained
- 1/4 cup minced onion
- 2 tbsp mayonnaise
- 1 tsp soy sauce
- 1/4 tsp garlic powder
- 1/4 tsp pepper
- 1 large whole wheat tortilla
- 4 lettuce leaves

INSTRUCTIONS

- Combine diced chicken, celery, onion, and oranges.
- Mix in mayo, soy sauce, garlic powder, and pepper.
- Place lettuce on tortilla and spoon in filling.
- Roll and serve chilled.

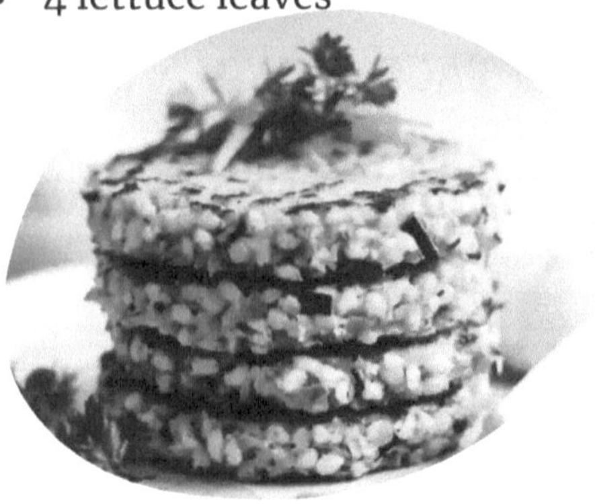

22. DELICIOUS MILLET CAKES

Crispy millet cakes with fresh herbs.

Nutrition: 250 kcal, 9g protein, 7g fat, 38g carbs, 270mg sodium

INGREDIENTS

- 1 tbsp olive oil
- 1/4 cup chopped onion
- 1 cup millet
- 1 clove garlic, minced
- 3 1/2 cups water
- 1/2 tsp salt
- 1/3 cup shredded zucchini
- 1/3 cup shredded carrot
- 1/3 cup grated Parmesan
- 1 tsp thyme
- 1 tsp lemon zest
- 1/4 tsp pepper

INSTRUCTIONS

- Cook onion and garlic in oil.
- Add millet, water, and salt; simmer 20 minutes.
- Stir in vegetables, cheese, thyme, zest, and pepper.
- Cool, form patties, and cook on a nonstick skillet 4 minutes per side.

23. QUESADILLAS & CILANTRO-YOGURT DIP

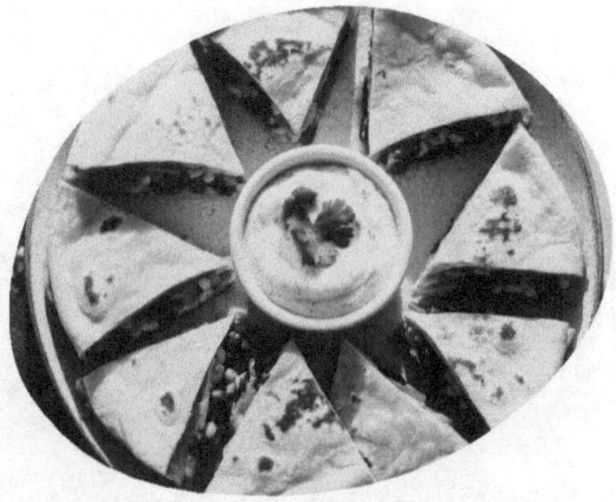

Cheesy quesadillas with yogurt dip.

Nutrition: 290 kcal, 16g protein, 8g fat, 34g carbs, 300mg sodium

INGREDIENTS

- 1 cup black beans
- ½ cup corn
- ½ cup chopped bell pepper
- 1 cup low-fat cheese
- 6 corn tortillas
- 2 tbsp chopped cilantro
- 1 shredded carrot
- Dip: 1 cup yogurt, 2 tbsp cilantro, juice of ½ lime

INSTRUCTIONS

- Assemble beans, corn, cheese, cilantro, and carrots between tortillas.
- Cook on skillet until cheese melts and tortillas are golden.
- Mix yogurt, cilantro, and lime juice for dip.
- Serve warm wedges with dip.

24. ROAST CHICKEN DAHL CURRY

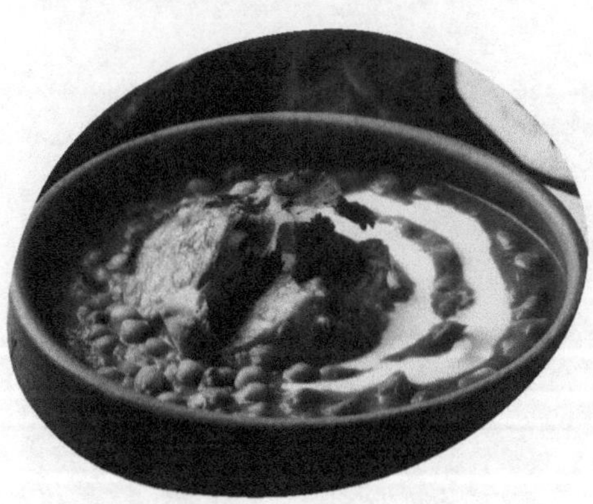

Chicken and lentils in light curry.

Nutrition: 310 kcal, 30g protein, 7g fat, 28g carbs, 290mg sodium

INGREDIENTS

- 1½ tsp canola oil
- 1 small onion, minced
- 2 tsp curry powder
- 1 can (15 oz) lentils, rinsed
- 1 can (14 oz) diced tomatoes
- 4 cups roasted chicken, diced
- ¼ tsp salt
- ¼ cup low-fat plain yogurt

INSTRUCTIONS

- Heat oil, sauté onion 3 minutes, and stir in curry powder.
- Add lentils, tomatoes, and chicken.
- Simmer until heated through.
- Remove from heat, stir in yogurt, and serve warm.

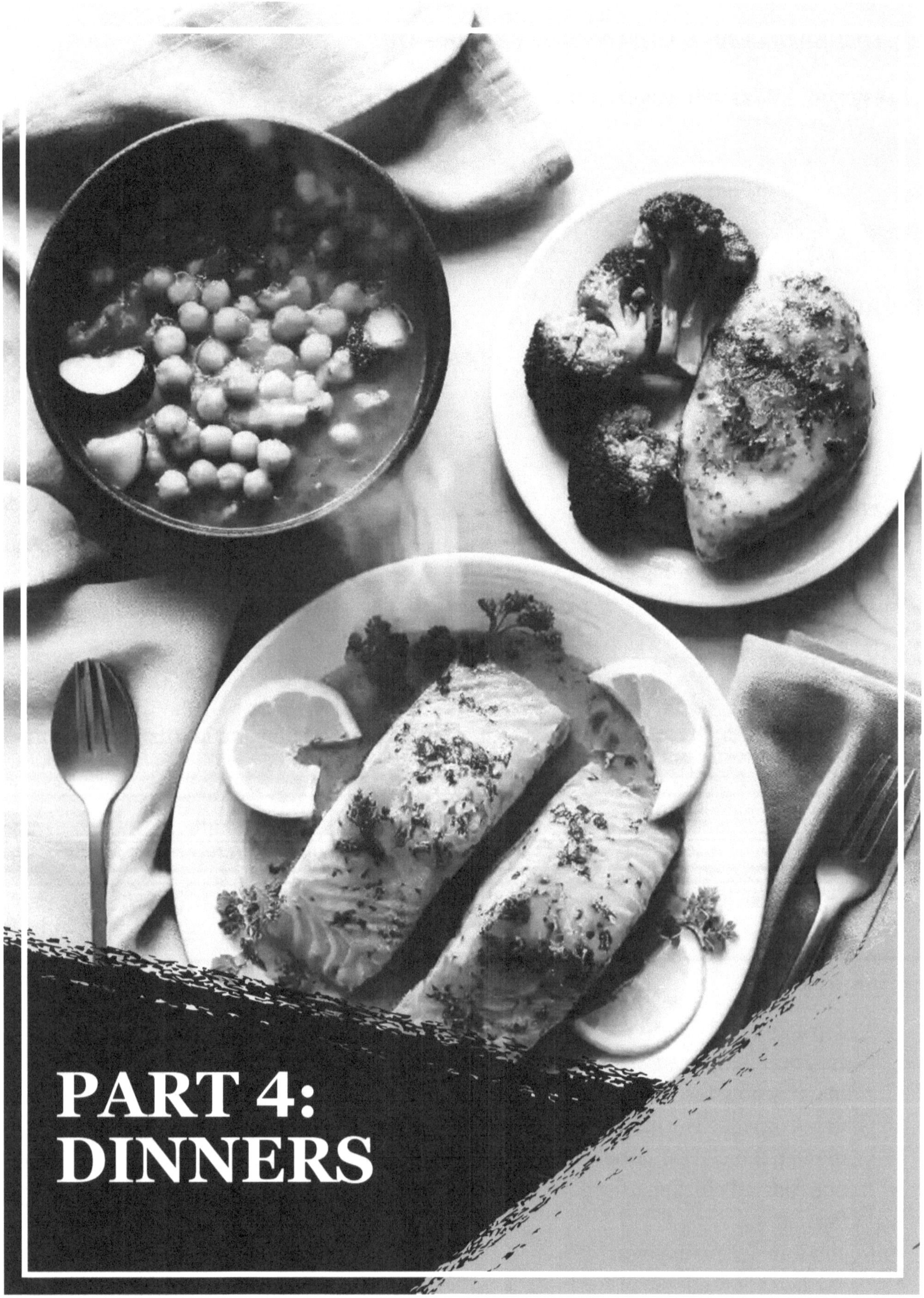

PART 4: DINNERS

1. LEMON GARLIC BAKED SALMON

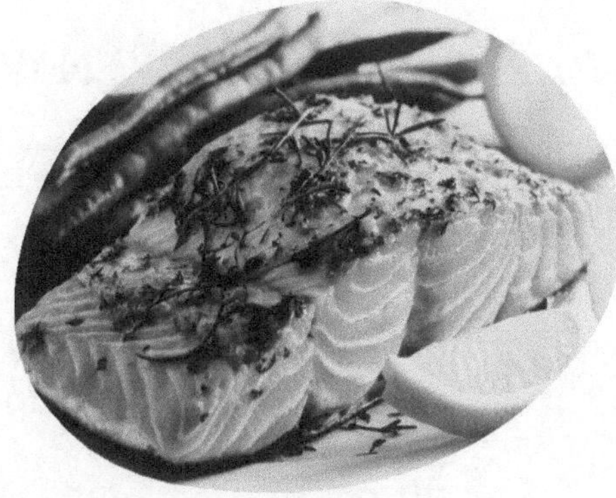

Flaky, bright, and full of heart-healthy omega-3s.

Nutrition: 285 kcal, 27g protein, 15g fat, 3g carbs, 130mg sodium

INGREDIENTS

- 4 salmon fillets
- 2 tbsp olive oil
- 2 cloves garlic, minced
- 1 tbsp lemon juice
- 1 tsp parsley
- 1 tsp black pepper

INSTRUCTIONS

- Preheat oven to 375°F.
- Brush olive oil over salmon.
- Mix garlic, lemon juice, and parsley, then spread on fillets.
- Season with black pepper.
- Bake for 15–18 minutes until fish flakes easily with a fork.
- Serve with steamed green beans or brown rice.

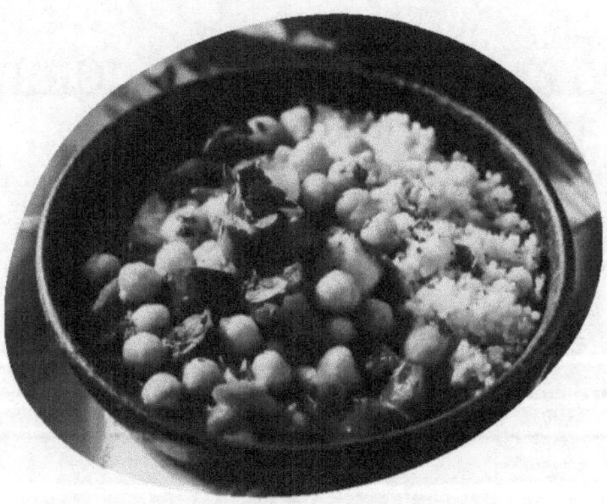

2. MEDITERRANEAN CHICKPEA STEW

A hearty vegetarian dish rich in fiber and antioxidants.

Nutrition: 240 kcal, 9g protein, 8g fat, 32g carbs, 180mg sodium

INGREDIENTS

- 1 tbsp olive oil
- 1 onion, chopped
- 2 cups cooked chickpeas
- 1 can diced tomatoes
- 1 zucchini, chopped
- 1 tsp cumin
- 1 tsp oregano

INSTRUCTIONS

- Heat olive oil in a saucepan.
- Add chopped onion and cook until soft.
- Stir in chickpeas, tomatoes, and zucchini.
- Season with cumin and oregano.
- Simmer uncovered for 15 minutes until thickened.
- Serve hot with cooked couscous or quinoa.

3. GARLIC HERB CHICKEN WITH SPINACH

Tender, juicy chicken in a simple herbal glaze.

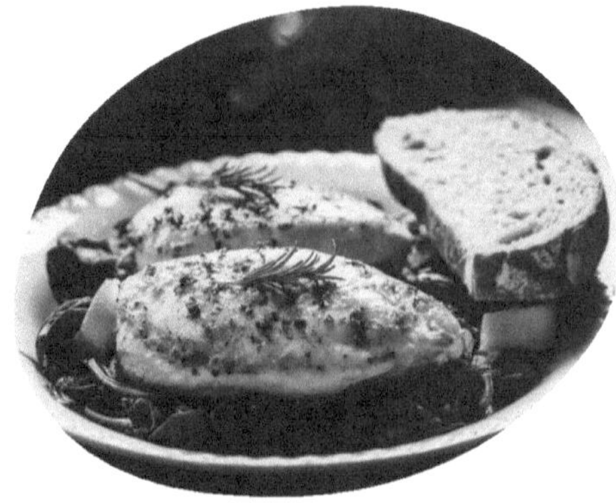

Nutrition: 230 kcal, 31g protein, 9g fat, 2g carbs, 140mg sodium

INGREDIENTS

- 2 boneless chicken breasts
- 1 tbsp olive oil
- 2 cloves garlic, minced
- 2 cups baby spinach
- ½ tsp thyme
- Juice of ½ lemon

INSTRUCTIONS

- Warm olive oil in a skillet.
- Add garlic and chicken breasts. Cook 5 minutes on each side.
- Add thyme and lemon juice. Stir to coat.
- Add spinach and cover for 2 minutes until wilted.
- Serve hot with a slice of whole-grain bread.

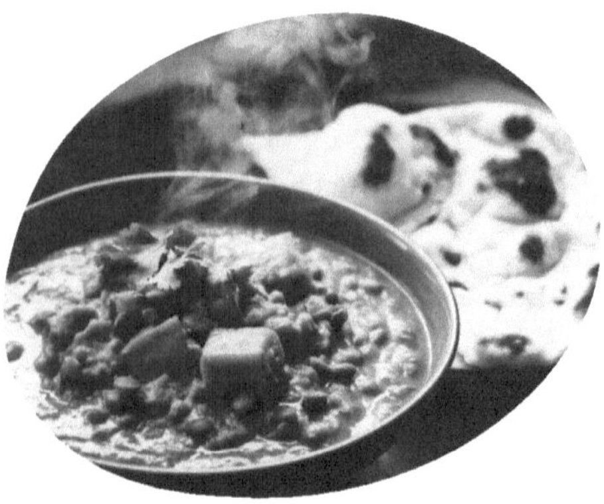

4. SWEET POTATO AND LENTIL CURRY

Comforting, mild, and rich in plant protein.

Nutrition: 270 kcal, 12g protein, 6g fat, 42g carbs, 160mg sodium

INGREDIENTS

- 1 tbsp olive oil
- 1 onion, diced
- 1 cup red lentils
- 1 cup cubed sweet potato
- 2 cups low-sodium vegetable broth
- 1 tsp turmeric
- ½ tsp chili powder

INSTRUCTIONS

- Sauté onion in olive oil until translucent.
- Add lentils, sweet potato, and broth.
- Stir in turmeric and chili powder.
- Cover and simmer for 25 minutes until thick and soft.
- Serve warm with brown rice or naan

5. BAKED COD WITH TOMATOES

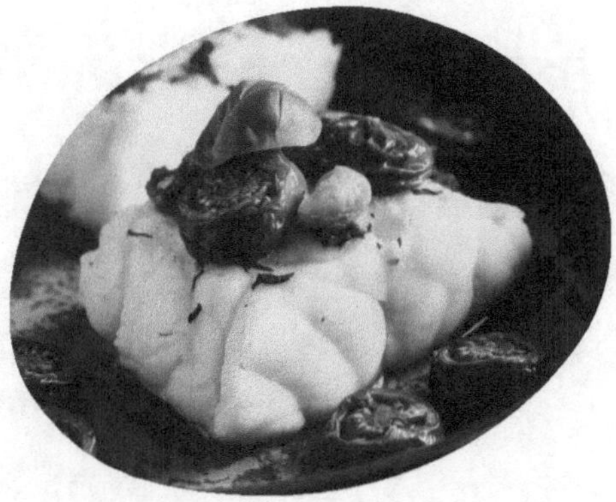

Light and full of Mediterranean flavor.

Nutrition: 190 kcal, 26g protein, 7g fat, 4g carbs, 120mg sodium

INGREDIENTS

- 4 cod fillets
- 1 tbsp olive oil
- 1 cup cherry tomatoes, halved
- 2 cloves garlic, minced
- ½ tsp basil
- ½ tsp black pepper

INSTRUCTIONS

- Preheat oven to 375°F.
- Place cod in a shallow baking dish.
- Top with tomatoes, garlic, and basil.
- Drizzle olive oil evenly over fish.
- Sprinkle with black pepper.
- Bake for 15 minutes or until fish flakes easily.

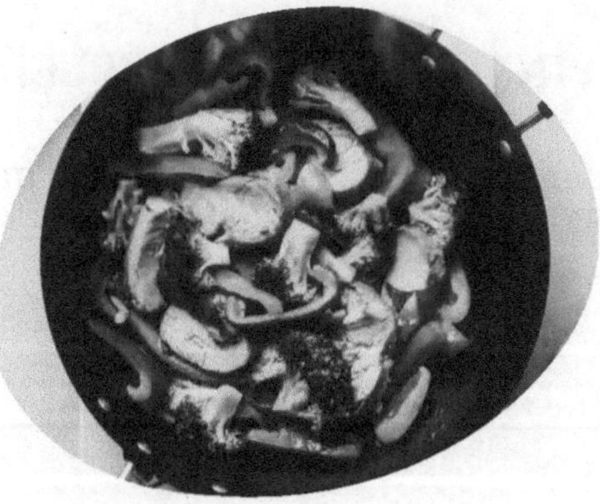

6. TURKEY AND VEGGIE STIR-FRY

Quick, colorful, and packed with lean protein.

Nutrition: 260 kcal, 25g protein, 9g fat, 14g carbs, 180mg sodium

INGREDIENTS

- 1 tbsp sesame oil
- 1 cup ground turkey
- 1 bell pepper, sliced
- 1 cup broccoli florets
- 2 tbsp low-sodium soy sauce
- 1 tsp grated ginger

INSTRUCTIONS

- Warm sesame oil in a skillet or wok.
- Add turkey and cook until browned.
- Add bell pepper, broccoli, and ginger.
- Stir-fry for 5 minutes until vegetables are tender.
- Pour soy sauce and toss well.
- Serve immediately over brown rice.

7. HERB AND LEMON CHICKEN QUINOA BOWL

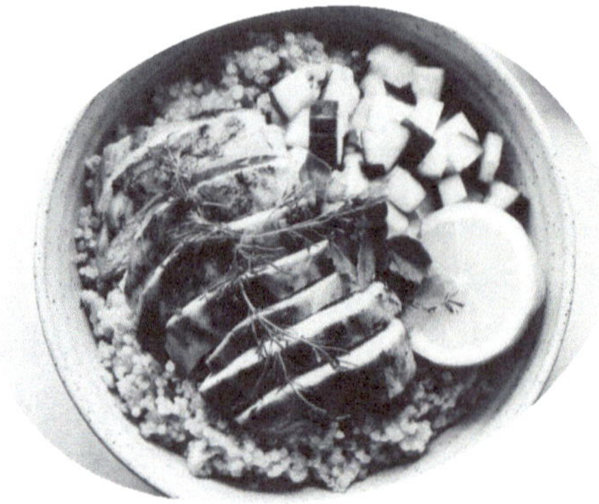

Fresh, light, and perfect for a balanced dinner.

Nutrition: 295 kcal, 28g protein, 9g fat, 22g carbs, 150mg sodium

INGREDIENTS

- 1 chicken breast, grilled
- 1 cup cooked quinoa
- ½ cup cucumber, diced
- 1 tbsp olive oil
- 1 tsp lemon juice
- ¼ tsp oregano

INSTRUCTIONS

- Toss quinoa with olive oil, lemon juice, and oregano.
- Add diced cucumber and mix gently.
- Slice grilled chicken into strips.
- Arrange over quinoa and serve warm or chilled.

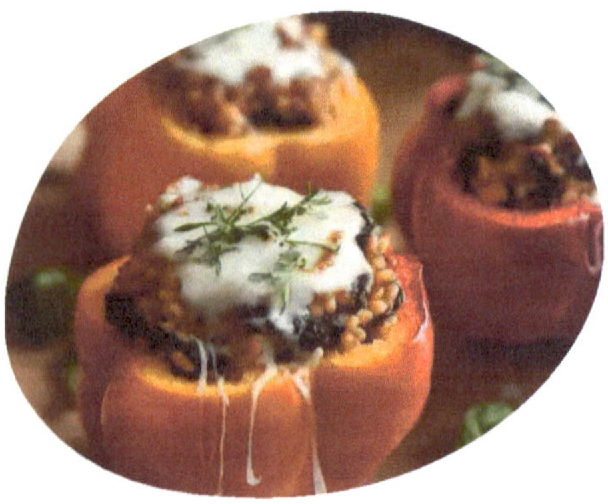

8. CREAMY SPINACH STUFFED PEPPERS

A colorful, cheesy meal rich in potassium and calcium.

Nutrition: 210 kcal, 8g protein, 7g fat, 28g carbs, 130mg sodium

INGREDIENTS

- 2 bell peppers, halved
- 1 cup cooked brown rice
- 1 cup spinach, chopped
- ¼ cup low-fat ricotta
- ½ tsp garlic powder
- 1 tsp olive oil

INSTRUCTIONS

- Preheat oven to 375°F.
- Mix rice, spinach, ricotta, and garlic powder in a bowl.
- Stuff the pepper halves with the mixture.
- Drizzle olive oil on top.
- Bake 20 minutes until peppers are tender.
- Serve warm.

9. SALMON AND ASPARAGUS FOIL PACKETS

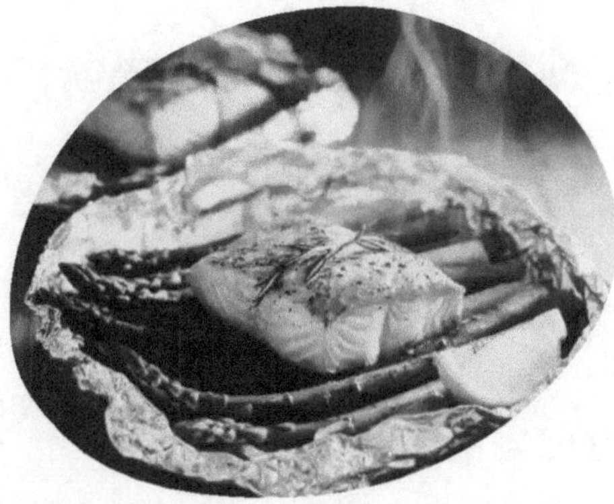

Simple, moist, and easy cleanup for busy evenings.

Nutrition: 285 kcal, 27g protein, 15g fat, 3g carbs, 130mg sodium

INGREDIENTS

- 2 salmon fillets
- 1 cup asparagus spears
- 1 tbsp olive oil
- 1 tsp dill
- Juice of 1/2 lemon
- 1/4 tsp black pepper

INSTRUCTIONS

- Preheat oven to 400°F.
- Place salmon and asparagus on foil.
- Drizzle olive oil and lemon juice over both.
- Sprinkle with dill and pepper.
- Seal the foil tightly and bake for 18 minutes.
- Open carefully and serve immediately.

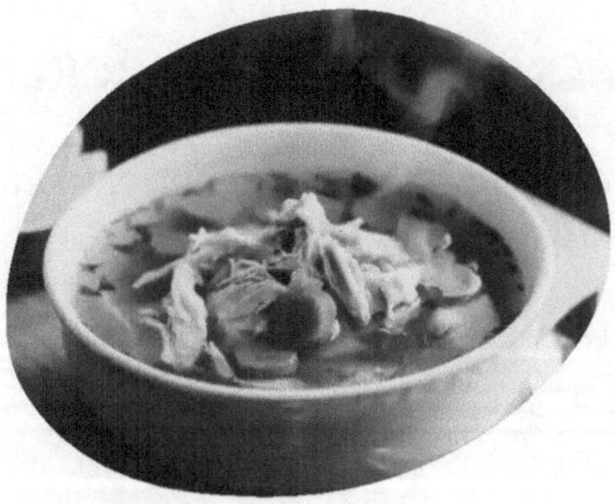

10. CHICKEN AND VEGETABLE SOUP

A cozy, soothing bowl perfect for gentle digestion.

Nutrition: 180 kcal, 22g protein, 6g fat, 9g carbs, 140mg sodium

INGREDIENTS

- 1 tsp olive oil
- 1/2 cup onion, diced
- 1 carrot, sliced
- 1 cup cooked chicken breast, shredded
- 2 cups low-sodium broth
- 1/4 tsp thyme
- 1/4 tsp black pepper

INSTRUCTIONS

- Heat olive oil in a saucepan.
- Add onion and carrot and cook for 4 minutes.
- Pour in the broth and season with thyme and pepper.
- Stir in the shredded chicken.
- Simmer 15 minutes until vegetables are soft.
- Serve warm in bowls.

11. MUSHROOM BARLEY RISOTTO

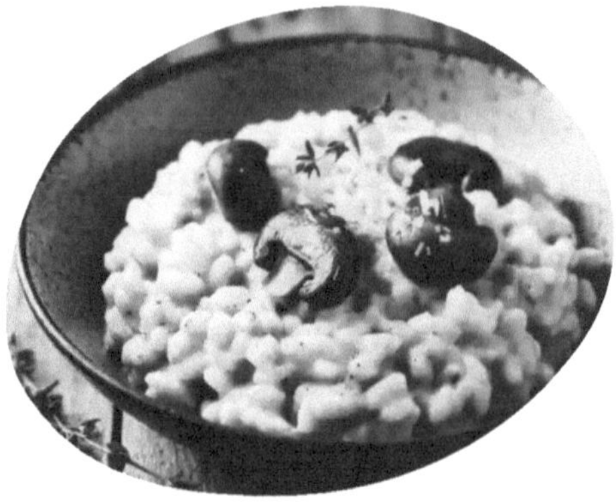

Creamy, savory, and naturally low in sodium.

Nutrition: 245 kcal, 9g protein, 8g fat, 34g carbs, 155mg sodium

INGREDIENTS

- 1 tbsp olive oil
- 1 cup mushrooms, sliced
- ½ cup pearl barley
- 2 cups low-sodium vegetable broth
- ¼ cup grated parmesan cheese
- ½ tsp dried thyme

INSTRUCTIONS

- Warm olive oil in a skillet.
- Add mushrooms and cook until golden brown.
- Stir in barley and toast lightly for 1 minute.
- Pour broth gradually, stirring until absorbed.
- Mix in parmesan and thyme before serving.
- Serve warm with a green salad.

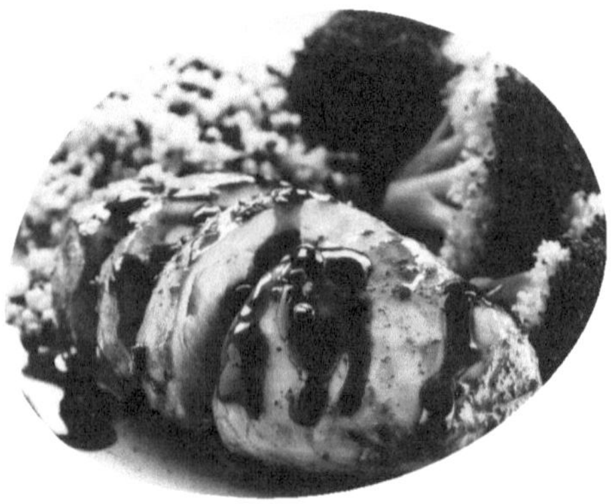

12. BALSAMIC GLAZED CHICKEN

Sweet, tangy, and rich in antioxidants

Nutrition: 240 kcal, 29g protein, 8g fat, 8g carbs, 135mg sodium

INGREDIENTS

- 2 boneless chicken breasts
- 1 tbsp olive oil
- 2 tbsp balsamic vinegar
- 1 tsp honey
- 1 garlic clove, minced
- ¼ tsp black pepper

INSTRUCTIONS

- Heat olive oil in a skillet.
- Add chicken and cook until golden on both sides.
- Mix vinegar, honey, and garlic in a small bowl.
- Pour sauce over chicken and simmer 5 minutes.
- Serve hot with steamed broccoli or quinoa.

13. LENTIL AND SPINACH SOUP

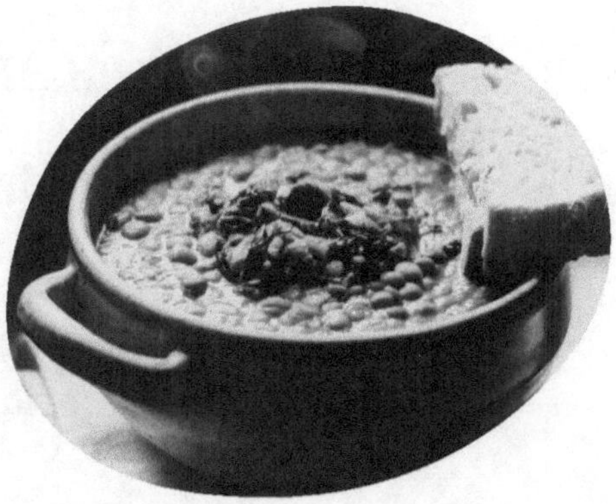

Simple, hearty, and full of plant-based protein.

Nutrition: 220 kcal, 12g protein, 4g fat, 34g carbs, 125mg sodium

INGREDIENTS

- 1 tbsp olive oil
- ½ onion, diced
- 1 cup dry lentils
- 3 cups low-sodium broth
- 1 cup spinach, chopped
- ¼ tsp cumin
- ¼ tsp black pepper

INSTRUCTIONS

- Sauté onion in olive oil until soft.
- Add lentils, broth, and seasonings.
- Simmer 30 minutes until lentils are tender.
- Stir in spinach and cook for 2 more minutes.
- Serve hot with a slice of whole-grain bread.

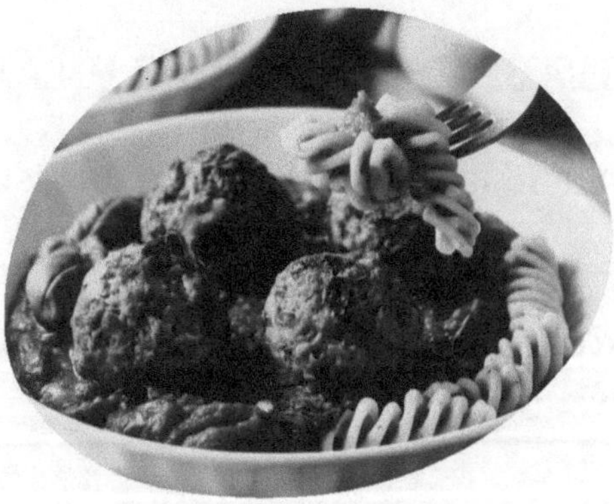

14. TURKEY MEATBALLS WITH TOMATO BASIL SAUCE

Tender and lean with a rich tomato flavor.

Nutrition: 260 kcal, 27g protein, 8g fat, 12g carbs, 150mg sodium

INGREDIENTS

- 1 lb ground turkey
- 1 egg
- 2 tbsp oats
- 1 tsp basil
- 1 can no-salt diced tomatoes
- 1 tsp olive oil

INSTRUCTIONS

- Preheat oven to 375°F.
- Mix turkey, egg, oats, and basil in a bowl.
- Form into small meatballs.
- Heat olive oil in a skillet and brown the meatballs.
- Add diced tomatoes and simmer 20 minutes.
- Serve with whole-wheat pasta or roasted vegetables.

15. BAKED TILAPIA WITH HERBS

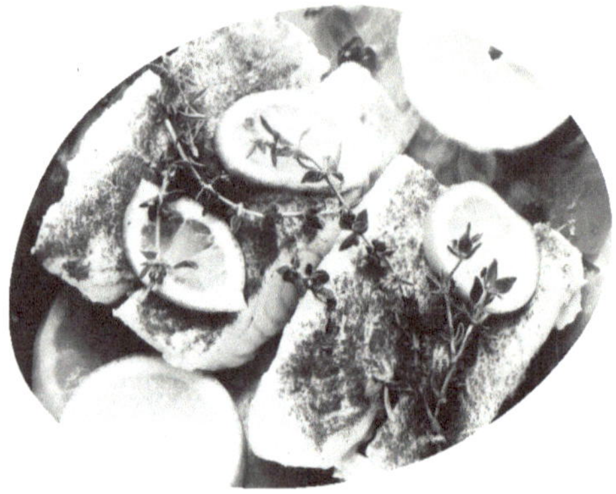

Quick, flavorful, and heart-healthy for any night.

Nutrition: 180 kcal, 26g protein, 6g fat, 2g carbs, 120mg sodium

INGREDIENTS

- 4 tilapia fillets
- 1 tbsp olive oil
- 1/2 tsp thyme
- 1/2 tsp paprika
- 1 tsp lemon juice
- 1/4 tsp black pepper

INSTRUCTIONS

- Preheat oven to 375°F.
- Place tilapia on a lined baking tray.
- Brush fillets with olive oil and lemon juice.
- Sprinkle thyme, paprika, and black pepper on top.
- Bake 12–15 minutes until fish flakes easily.
- Serve with steamed vegetables.

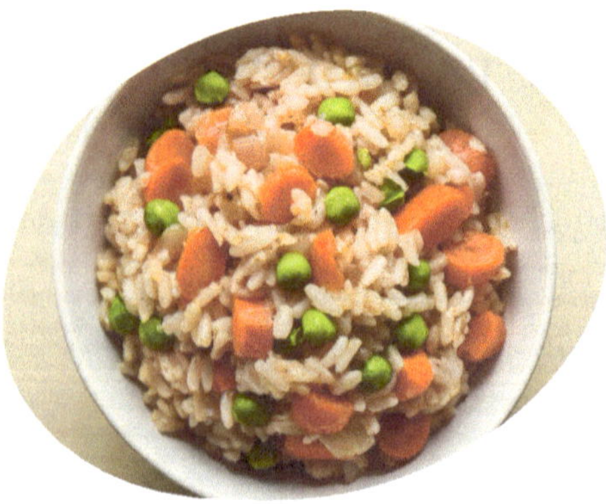

16. VEGETABLE BROWN RICE PILAF

Colorful, fiber-rich, and ideal as a side or main dish.

Nutrition: 210 kcal, 5g protein, 7g fat, 33g carbs, 115mg sodium

INGREDIENTS

- 1 cup brown rice, cooked
- 1 tbsp olive oil
- 1 carrot, diced
- 1/2 cup peas
- 1/4 cup onion, chopped
- 1/4 tsp turmeric
- 1/4 tsp pepper

INSTRUCTIONS

- Heat olive oil in a skillet.
- Add onion and carrot and sauté for 4 minutes.
- Add cooked rice, peas, and turmeric.
- Stir until all ingredients are evenly mixed.
- Cook 3 minutes on low heat.
- Serve warm with grilled fish or tofu.

17. SHRIMP AND SPINACH STIR-FRY

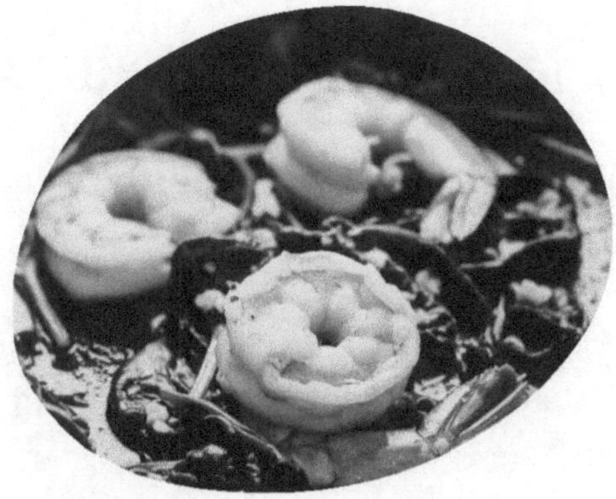

Light, quick, and full of omega-3s.

Nutrition: 200 kcal, 25g protein, 8g fat, 3g carbs, 170mg sodium

INGREDIENTS

- 1 tbsp olive oil
- ½ lb shrimp, peeled
- 2 cups baby spinach
- 1 garlic clove, minced
- 1 tsp lemon juice
- ¼ tsp black pepper

INSTRUCTIONS

- Heat olive oil in a skillet.
- Add shrimp and garlic, cooking for 2–3 minutes.
- Add spinach and stir until wilted.
- Drizzle lemon juice and sprinkle pepper.
- Cook 1 more minute and serve immediately.

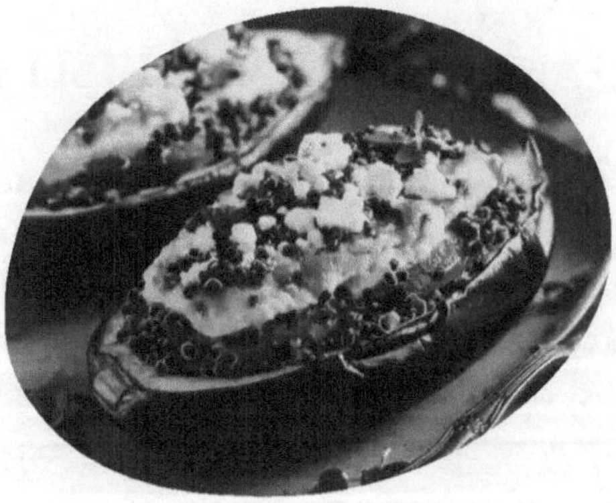

18. STUFFED EGGPLANT WITH QUINOA

Soft, savory, and packed with plant protein.

Nutrition: 230 kcal, 8g protein, 9g fat, 29g carbs, 140mg sodium

INGREDIENTS

- 1 large eggplant, halved
- 1 cup cooked quinoa
- ½ cup diced tomato
- 1 tbsp olive oil
- 1 tsp oregano
- 2 tbsp feta cheese

INSTRUCTIONS

- Preheat oven to 375°F.
- Scoop out eggplant flesh and chop finely.
- Sauté chopped eggplant in olive oil.
- Mix with quinoa, tomato, and oregano.
- Spoon filling into shells and top with feta.
- Bake 20 minutes until tender.

19. LEMON HERB CHICKEN AND BROCCOLI

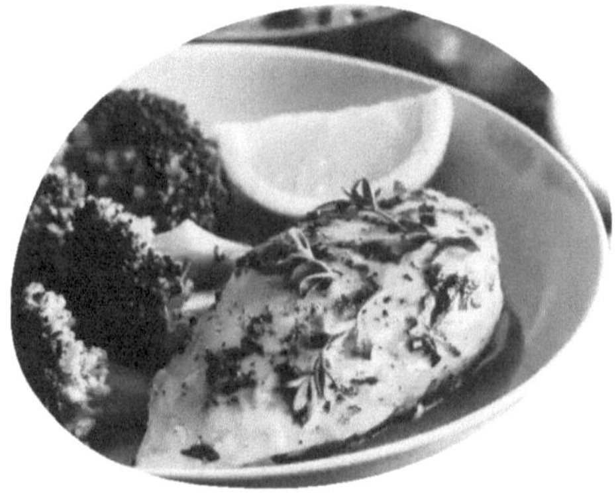

Simple, bright, and great for circulation.

Nutrition: 225 kcal, 29g protein, 8g fat, 5g carbs, 135mg sodium

INGREDIENTS

- 2 chicken breasts
- 1 tbsp olive oil
- 1 cup broccoli florets
- 1 tbsp lemon juice
- ½ tsp garlic powder
- ¼ tsp black pepper

INSTRUCTIONS

- Heat olive oil in a skillet.
- Add chicken and cook until lightly golden.
- Add broccoli and lemon juice.
- Sprinkle garlic powder and pepper.
- Cover and cook for 3 minutes.
- Serve warm.

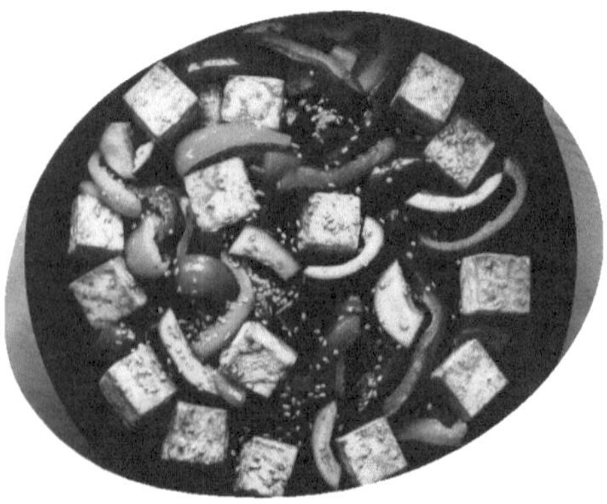

20. TOFU AND VEGETABLE SKILLET

A high-protein vegetarian meal rich in flavor.

Nutrition: 210 kcal, 12g protein, 11g fat, 15g carbs, 155mg sodium

INGREDIENTS

- Ingredients:
- 1 tbsp olive oil
- 1 cup firm tofu, cubed
- ½ cup bell peppers, chopped
- ½ cup zucchini, sliced
- 2 tbsp low-sodium soy sauce
- 1 tsp sesame seeds

INSTRUCTIONS

- Heat olive oil in a skillet.
- Add tofu cubes and cook until lightly golden.
- Add vegetables and cook 4 minutes.
- Pour soy sauce and sprinkle sesame seeds.
- Cook 2 more minutes and serve hot.

21. GARLIC SHRIMP WITH ZUCCHINI NOODLES

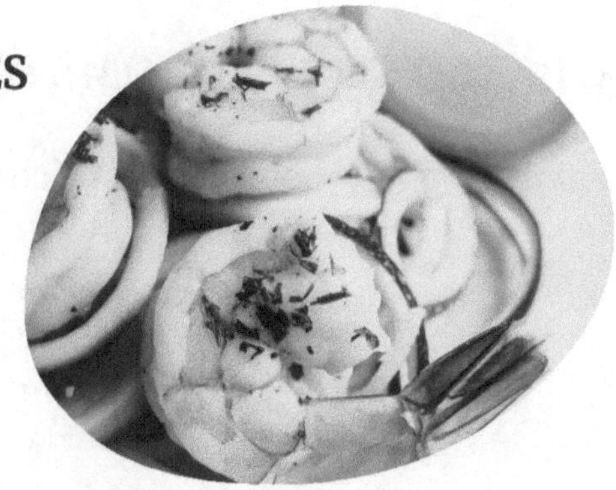

A light, low-carb twist on pasta night.

Nutrition: 205 kcal, 25g protein, 8g fat, 4g carbs, 140mg sodium

INGREDIENTS

- 1 tbsp olive oil
- ½ lb shrimp, peeled
- 2 cloves garlic, minced
- 2 medium zucchinis, spiralized
- 1 tbsp lemon juice
- ¼ tsp crushed red pepper

INSTRUCTIONS

- Warm olive oil in a skillet.
- Add shrimp and garlic and sauté for 3 minutes.
- Add zucchini noodles and toss gently.
- Pour in lemon juice and sprinkle red pepper.
- Cook 2 minutes until shrimp are pink.
- Serve immediately.

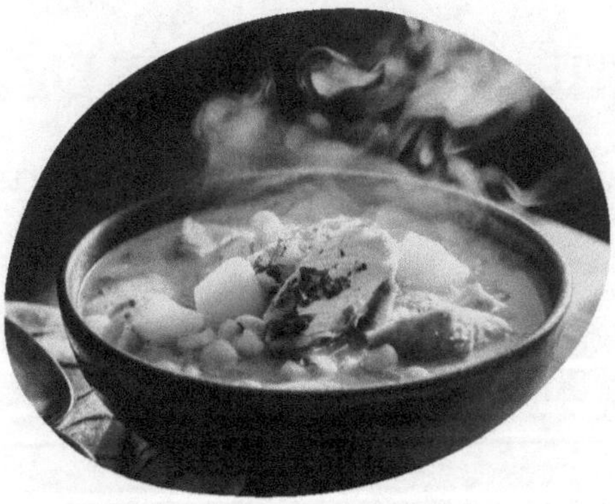

22. HEARTY CHICKEN AND SWEET CORN STEW

Comforting, creamy, and perfect for cool evenings.

Nutrition: 235 kcal, 25g protein, 6g fat, 21g carbs, 145mg sodium

INGREDIENTS

- 1 tsp olive oil
- 1 chicken breast, diced
- 1 small onion, chopped
- 1 cup corn kernels
- 1 cup diced potato
- 2 cups low-sodium chicken broth
- ¼ tsp thyme

INSTRUCTIONS

- Heat olive oil in a pot.
- Add chicken and onion, cooking until lightly golden.
- Add corn, potato, and broth.
- Season with thyme and stir well.
- Simmer 20 minutes until vegetables are tender.
- Serve warm in bowls.

23. BAKED STUFFED TOMATOES

A colorful, plant-based dinner rich in antioxidants.

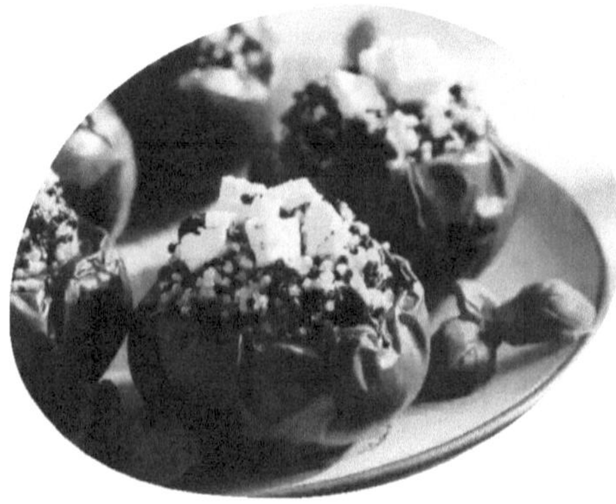

Nutrition: 285 kcal, 27g protein, 15g fat, 3g carbs, 130mg sodium

INGREDIENTS

- 4 large tomatoes
- 1 cup cooked quinoa
- 1/2 cup spinach, chopped
- 2 tbsp feta cheese
- 1 tsp olive oil
- 1/4 tsp black pepper

INSTRUCTIONS

- Preheat oven to 375°F.
- Cut tops off tomatoes and scoop out centers.
- Mix quinoa, spinach, feta, and pepper in a bowl.
- Stuff each tomato and drizzle olive oil on top.
- Bake for 15–18 minutes until tender.

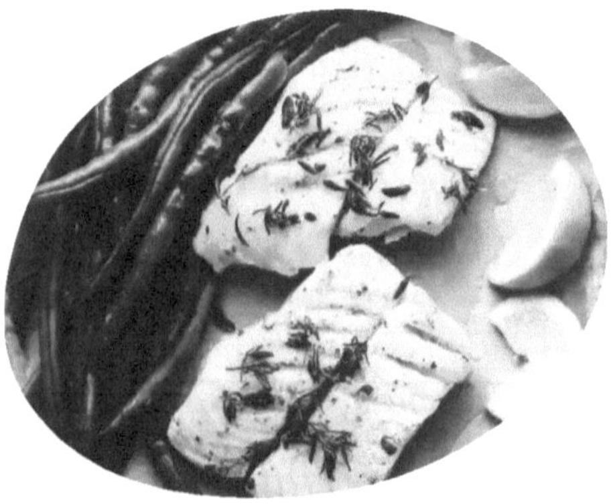

24. LEMON HERB TILAPIA WITH GREEN BEANS

A quick, protein-packed meal for healthy hearts.

Nutrition: 185 kcal, 26g protein, 6g fat, 3g carbs, 125mg sodium

INGREDIENTS

- 2 tilapia fillets
- 1 tbsp olive oil
- 1 cup green beans
- 1 tbsp lemon juice
- 1/2 tsp dill
- 1/4 tsp black pepper

INSTRUCTIONS

- Preheat oven to 375°F.
- Place tilapia on foil and drizzle with olive oil.
- Add green beans beside the fish.
- Sprinkle dill, pepper, and lemon juice.
- Seal foil and bake for 15 minutes.
- Serve immediately.

25. VEGGIE AND BROWN RICE CASSEROLE

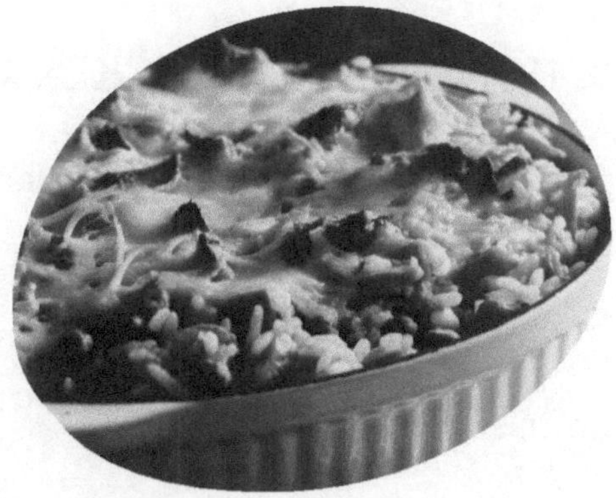

Comforting and full of fiber for long-lasting energy.

Nutrition: 225 kcal, 6g protein, 8g fat, 33g carbs, 150mg sodium

INGREDIENTS

- 1 tbsp olive oil
- 1 cup cooked brown rice
- ½ cup peas
- ½ cup chopped carrots
- ¼ cup low-fat cheddar cheese
- ¼ tsp black pepper

INSTRUCTIONS

- Preheat oven to 350°F.
- Sauté carrots and peas in olive oil for 4 minutes.
- Mix with brown rice and pepper.
- Transfer to a baking dish and sprinkle cheese on top.
- Bake for 10 minutes until warm and melted.
- Serve immediately.

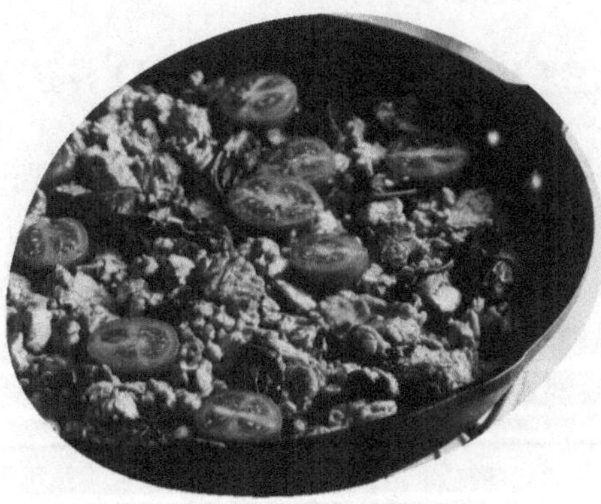

26. TURKEY AND SPINACH SKILLET

A high-protein one-pan dinner that's easy to chew.

Nutrition: 235 kcal, 28g protein, 9g fat, 5g carbs, 160mg sodium

INGREDIENTS

- 1 tbsp olive oil
- ½ lb lean ground turkey
- 2 cups spinach, chopped
- ½ cup diced tomato
- 1 tsp garlic powder
- ¼ tsp black pepper

INSTRUCTIONS

- Heat olive oil in skillet.
- Add turkey and cook until browned.
- Add spinach, tomato, and garlic powder.
- Stir and cook 3–4 minutes.
- Season with pepper and serve warm.

27. HONEY DIJON CHICKEN WITH BROCCOLI

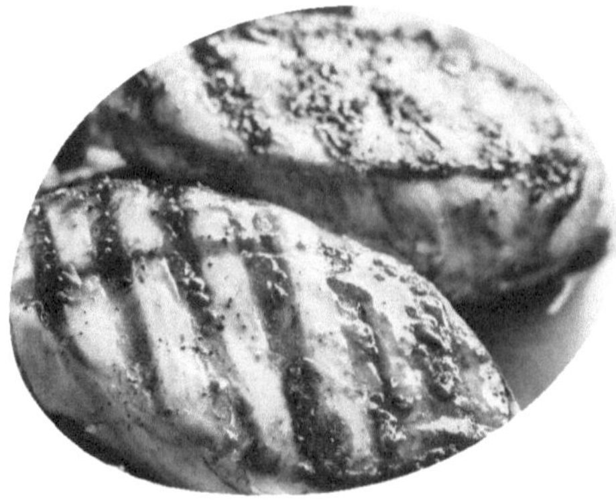

Sweet and savory with heart-smart flavors.

Nutrition: 240 kcal, 29g protein, 8g fat, 7g carbs, 135mg sodium

INGREDIENTS

- 2 chicken breasts
- 1 tbsp olive oil
- 1 tsp Dijon mustard
- 1 tsp honey
- 1 cup broccoli florets
- 1/4 tsp black pepper

INSTRUCTIONS

- Whisk mustard, honey, and olive oil together.
- Coat chicken with the mixture.
- Heat skillet and cook chicken 6 minutes each side.
- Add broccoli and pepper, cover, and steam 3 minutes.
- Serve hot.

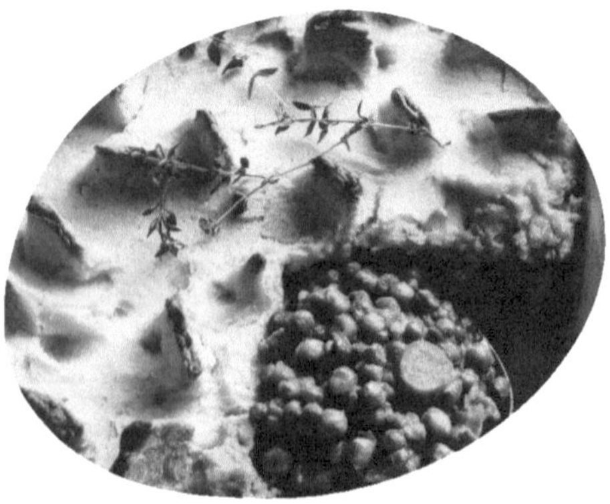

28. VEGETABLE LENTIL SHEPHERD'S PIE

A plant-based version of a classic comfort dish.

Nutrition: 260 kcal, 10g protein, 5g fat, 40g carbs, 150mg sodium

INGREDIENTS

- 1 cup cooked lentils
- 1 cup mashed sweet potato
- 1/2 cup peas
- 1/2 cup diced carrots
- 1 tsp olive oil
- 1/4 tsp thyme

INSTRUCTIONS

- Preheat oven to 375°F.
- Sauté peas and carrots in olive oil.
- Mix with lentils and thyme.
- Spread mixture in a baking dish.
- Top with mashed sweet potatoes.
- Bake 20 minutes until lightly golden.
- Serve warm.

29. BROILED CITRUS HERB SALMON

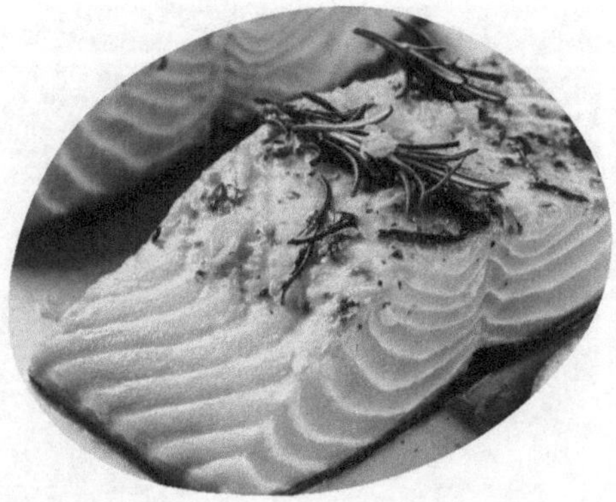

Zesty and rich in omega-3s for a healthy heart.

Nutrition: 280 kcal, 27g protein, 14g fat, 3g carbs, 125mg sodium

INGREDIENTS

- 2 salmon fillets
- 1 tbsp olive oil
- 1 tbsp orange juice
- 1 tsp lemon zest
- 1/2 tsp rosemary
- 1/4 tsp black pepper

INSTRUCTIONS

- Preheat broiler.
- Whisk oil, juice, zest, and rosemary.
- Brush mixture on salmon.
- Broil 6–8 minutes until fish flakes easily.
- Sprinkle with pepper and serve warm.

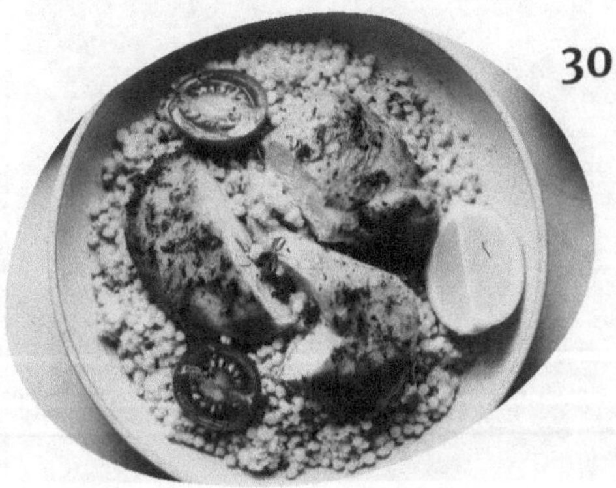

30. MEDITERRANEAN CHICKEN WITH COUSCOUS

Bright, balanced, and full of heart-healthy flavor.

Nutrition: 285 kcal, 29g protein, 8g fat, 23g carbs, 145mg sodium

INGREDIENTS

- 1 chicken breast, cubed
- 1 tbsp olive oil
- 1 cup cooked whole-wheat couscous
- 1/2 cup cherry tomatoes, halved
- 1 tsp oregano
- 1 tsp lemon juice

INSTRUCTIONS

- Heat olive oil in a pan.
- Add chicken and cook until golden.
- Stir in tomatoes, oregano, and lemon juice.
- Add couscous and toss until warmed.
- Serve immediately.

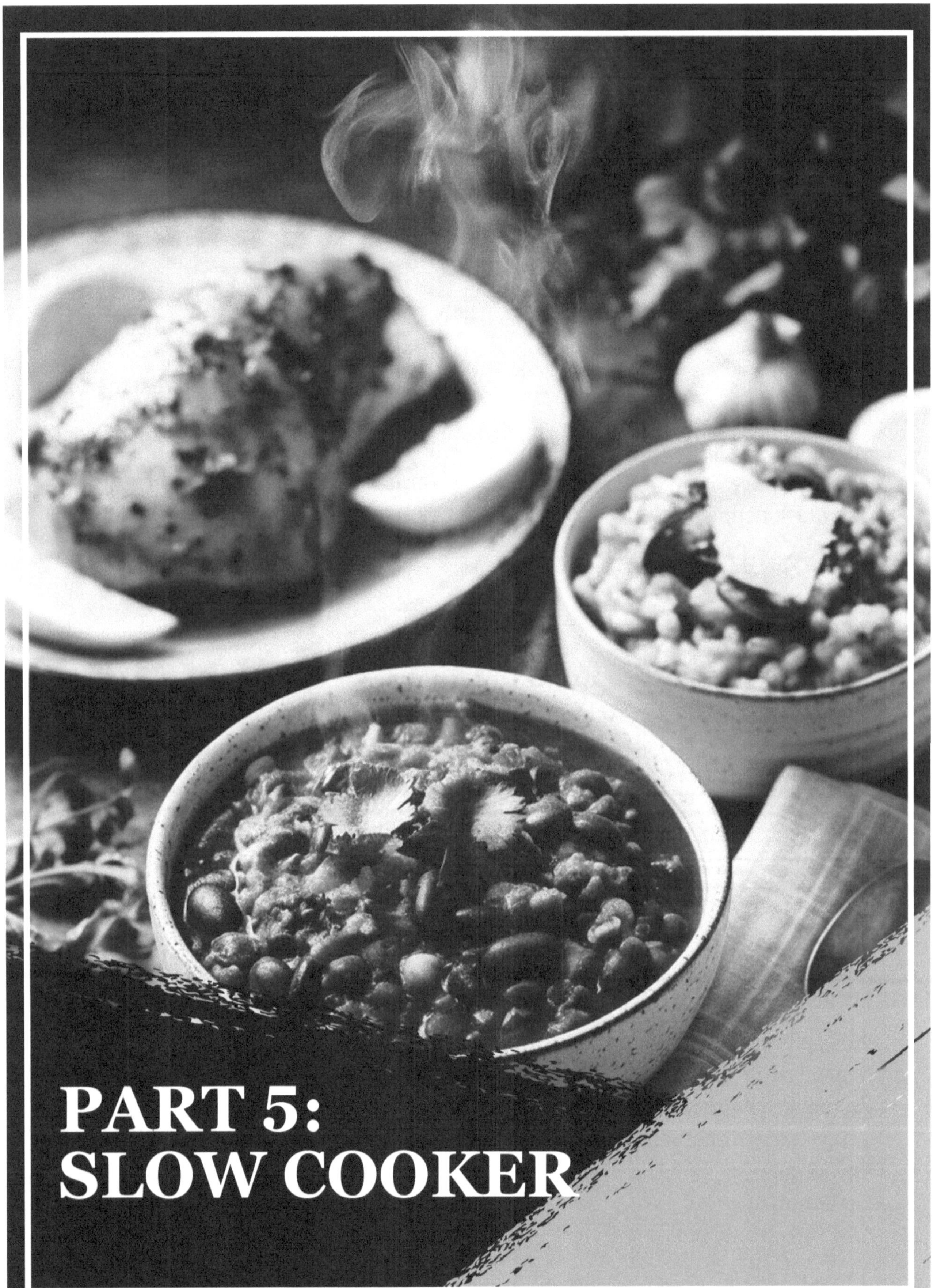

PART 5: SLOW COOKER

1. LEMON CROCK POT CHICKEN

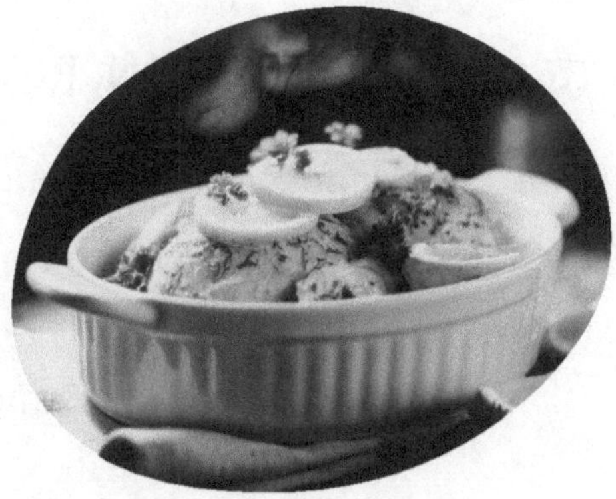

Tender, tangy, and heart-healthy with bright citrus flavor.

Nutrition: 210 kcal, 30g protein, 7g fat, 2g carbs, 240mg sodium.

INGREDIENTS

- 2 boneless skinless chicken breasts
- 1/4 cup low-sodium chicken broth
- 1/4 cup lemon juice
- 2 tbsp unsalted butter
- 1 tbsp Italian seasoning
- 3 garlic cloves, minced
- 1 tsp onion powder
- 1/2 tsp pepper

INSTRUCTIONS

- Season chicken with pepper and Italian seasoning.
- Brown lightly in butter and transfer to crock pot.
- Pour in broth, lemon juice, and garlic.
- Cook on low for 4 1/2 to 5 hours until tender.
- Serve warm with steamed vegetables.

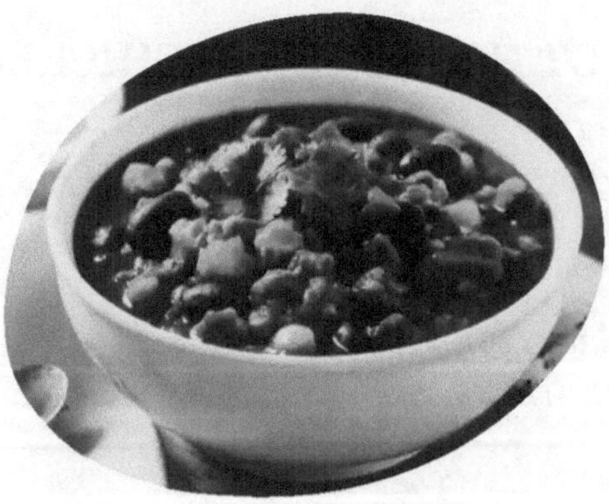

2. TURKEY CHILI

A hearty, low-fat chili that keeps sodium and cholesterol low.

Nutrition: 240 kcal, 27g protein, 6g fat, 21g carbs, 310mg sodium.

INGREDIENTS

- 1 lb lean ground turkey
- 1 medium onion, diced
- 1 bell pepper, chopped
- 1 can kidney beans, rinsed
- 1 can diced tomatoes
- 1 cup low-sodium chicken broth
- 1 tsp cumin
- 1 tsp chili powder
- 1/2 tsp oregano

INSTRUCTIONS

- Brown turkey in skillet, then place in crock pot with onion, bell pepper, beans, tomatoes, broth, and spices.
- Stir and cook on low for 6 to 7 hours.
- Serve hot with fresh spinach or a side salad.

3. CROCK POT CHICKEN, RICE & VEGGIE SOUP

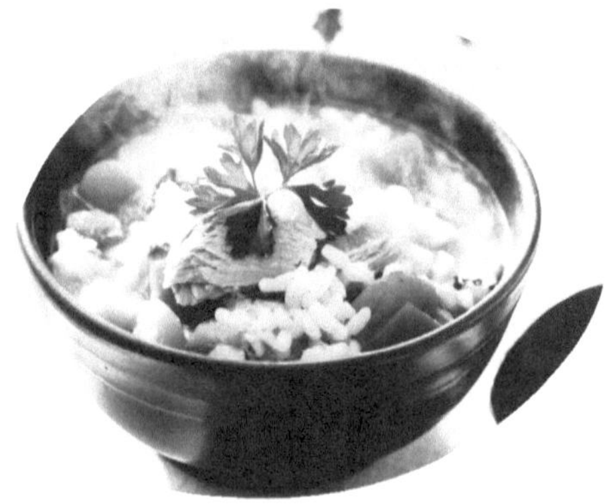

Gentle, nourishing, and easy to digest for seniors.

Nutrition: 190 kcal, 18g protein, 3g fat, 22g carbs, 180mg sodium.

INGREDIENTS

- 12 oz boneless chicken, diced
- 1 cup brown rice
- 2 cups mixed vegetables
- 4 cups low-sodium chicken broth
- 1/4 tsp black pepper

INSTRUCTIONS

- Place all ingredients into the slow cooker.
- Stir gently.
- Cook on high for 4 hours or until rice and vegetables are tender.
- Serve warm in bowls with parsley garnish.

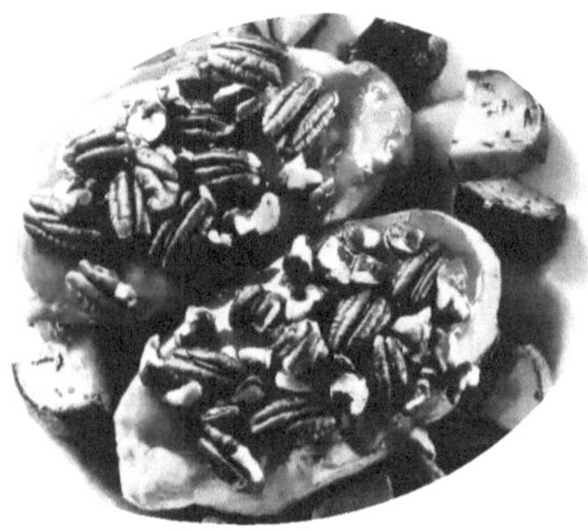

4. CROCK POT HONEY PECAN CHICKEN

Bright, balanced, and full of heart-healthy flavor.

Nutrition: 285 kcal, 29g protein, 8g fat, 23g carbs, 145mg sodium

INGREDIENTS

- 1 chicken breast, cubed
- 1 tbsp olive oil
- 1 cup cooked whole-wheat couscous
- 1/2 cup cherry tomatoes, halved
- 1 tsp oregano
- 1 tsp lemon juice

INSTRUCTIONS

- Brown chicken briefly in olive oil.
- Add all ingredients to the slow cooker and stir.
- Cook on low for 6 hours until chicken is soft and glazed.
- Garnish with parsley before serving.

5. SWEET & SOUR CROCK POT CHICKEN OVER BROWN RICE

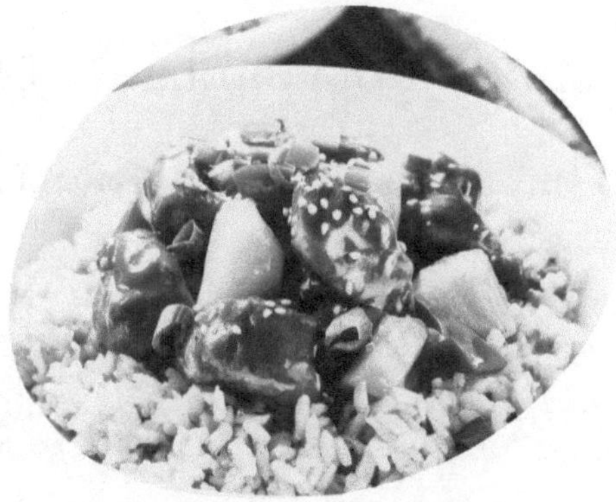

A balanced blend of sweet pineapple and tangy spice.

Nutrition: 260 kcal, 25g protein, 5g fat, 27g carbs, 230mg sodium.

INGREDIENTS

- 4 chicken breasts
- 1 onion, sliced
- 1 cup pineapple chunks
- 1 tbsp low-sodium soy sauce
- 2 tsp brown sugar
- ½ tsp ground ginger
- 3 tbsp cornstarch
- ¼ cup water
- 3 cups cooked brown rice

INSTRUCTIONS

- Layer onions and chicken in crock pot, add pineapple, soy sauce, sugar, and ginger.
- Cook on low for 6½ hours.
- Mix cornstarch and water, add to pot, and stir until thick.
- Serve over rice.

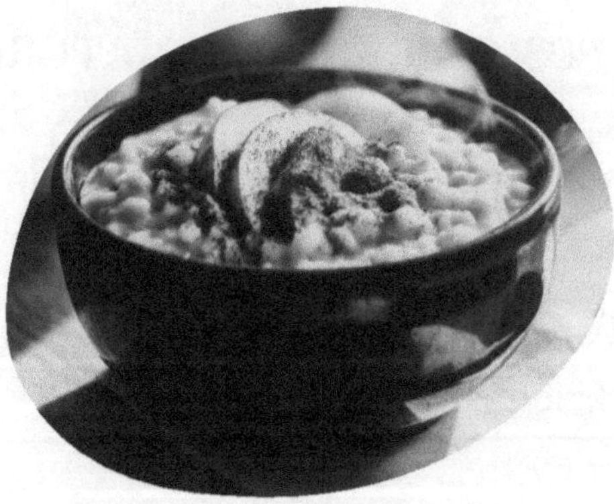

6. CROCK POT APPLE CINNAMON OATMEAL

A warm, naturally sweet breakfast packed with fiber.

Nutrition: 180 kcal, 4g protein, 2g fat, 38g carbs, 60mg sodium.

INGREDIENTS

- 1 apple, peeled and sliced
- ½ tsp cinnamon
- 2 tbsp brown sugar
- 1 cup rolled oats
- 2 cups water
- Dash salt

INSTRUCTIONS

- Place all ingredients in crock pot.
- Stir gently.
- Cover and cook on low for 8 hours.
- Stir before serving and top with fresh fruit or a drizzle of honey.

7. MUSHROOM BARLEY CROCK POT RISOTTO

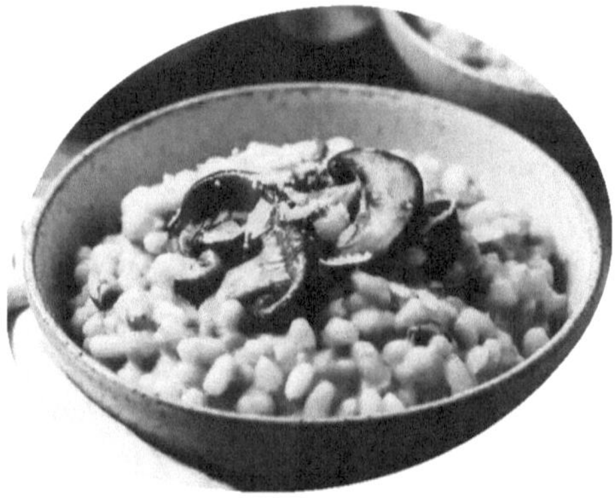

Creamy and rich in fiber, perfect for balanced digestion.

Nutrition: 215 kcal, 6g protein, 5g fat, 37g carbs, 170mg sodium

INGREDIENTS

- 1 tbsp olive oil
- 1 onion, chopped
- 1 cup mushrooms, sliced
- 1½ cups pearl barley
- 3 cups low-sodium broth
- 2 tbsp grated parmesan
- ½ tsp thyme

INSTRUCTIONS

- Sauté onion and mushrooms in oil.
- Add barley, thyme, and broth to crock pot.
- Cook on high for 3½ hours until soft.
- Stir in parmesan before serving.

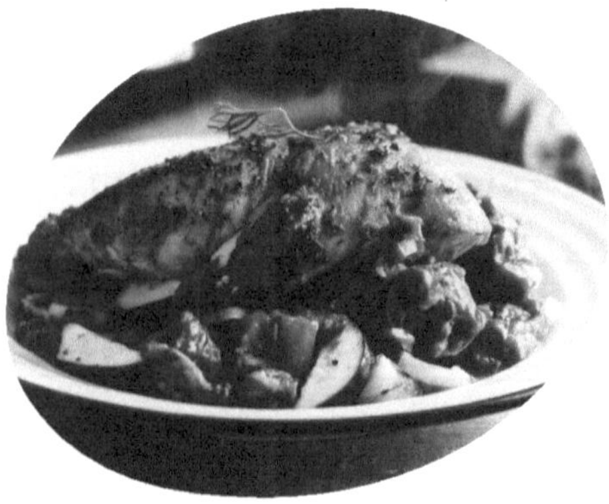

8. CROCK POT CHICKEN CACCIATORE

A light Italian-inspired dish rich in vegetables.

Nutrition: 225 kcal, 28g protein, 6g fat, 15g carbs, 260mg sodium.

INGREDIENTS

- 2 lb chicken breasts
- 2 zucchini, chopped
- 1 onion, sliced
- 1 jar low-sodium tomato sauce
- ½ tsp basil
- ½ tsp oregano

INSTRUCTIONS

- Add all ingredients to crock pot.
- Cover and cook on low for 7½ hours.
- Serve with whole-grain pasta or brown rice.

9. CROCK POT PEA & HAM SOUP

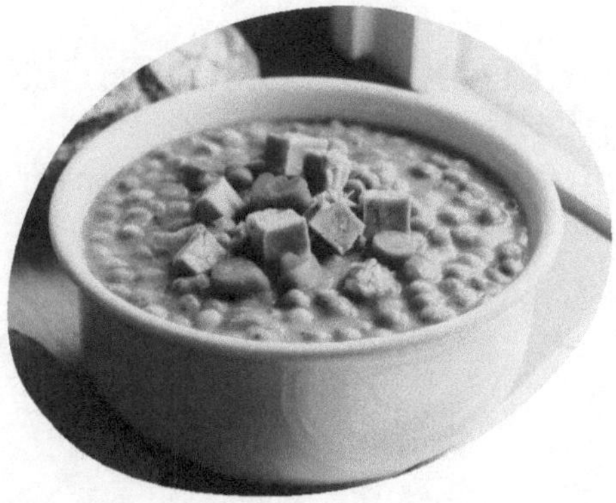

Comforting and high in fiber with reduced sodium.

Nutrition: 210 kcal, 16g protein, 4g fat, 28g carbs, 220mg sodium

INGREDIENTS

- 1 cup dried split peas
- 1 cup carrots, chopped
- 1 cup celery, sliced
- 1 onion, diced
- 1 cup cooked low-sodium ham
- 6 cups water
- 1/2 tsp seasoning blend

INSTRUCTIONS

- Combine all ingredients in crock pot.
- Stir and cook on high for 5 hours until peas are tender.
- Blend lightly for creamier texture.

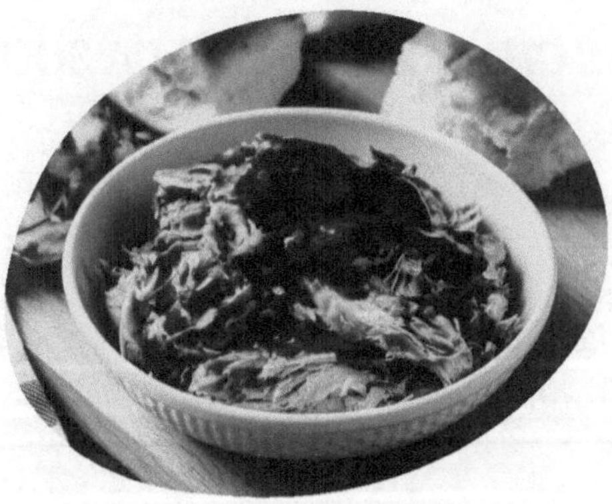

10. CROCK POT BARBEQUE CHICKEN

Tender shredded chicken with a smoky-sweet flavor.

Nutrition: 240 kcal, 29g protein, 5g fat, 18g carbs, 190mg sodium.

INGREDIENTS

- 4 boneless chicken breasts
- 3/4 cup ketchup
- 1 tbsp Worcestershire sauce
- 1 tsp lemon juice
- 1/2 tsp chili powder

INSTRUCTIONS

- Combine all ingredients in crock pot and mix.
- Cook on low for 7 1/2 hours.
- Shred chicken and serve on whole wheat buns or with rice.

11. CROCK POT PORK CHOPS WITH CREAMY SAUCE

Soft, savory, and easy to chew for tender appetites.

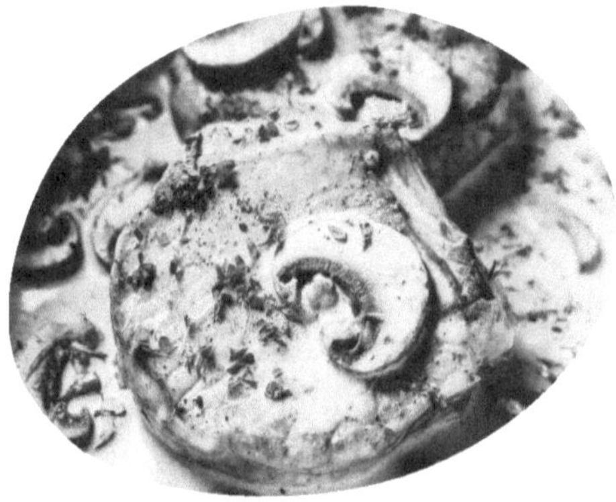

Nutrition: 235 kcal, 27g protein, 9g fat, 6g carbs, 210mg sodium.

INGREDIENTS

- 4 boneless pork chops
- 1 can low-sodium cream of mushroom soup
- ½ cup low-sodium chicken broth
- ¼ tsp black pepper

INSTRUCTIONS

- Place all ingredients in crock pot, cover, and cook on low for 7 hours until pork is tender.
- Serve with mashed sweet potatoes.

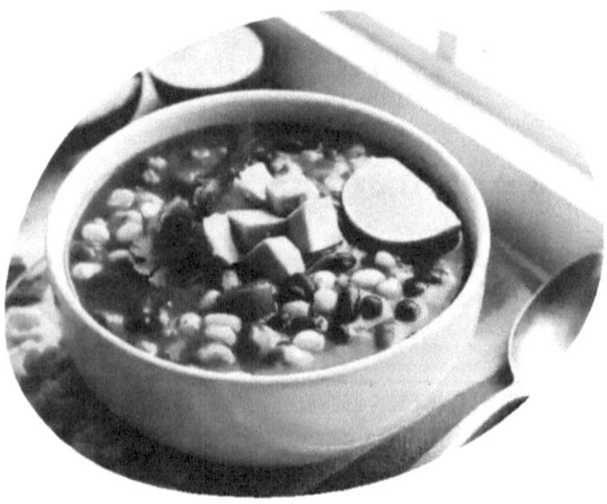

12. CROCK POT CHICKEN TORTILLA SOUP

Spiced and satisfying without heavy salt.

Nutrition: 200 kcal, 22g protein, 4g fat, 20g carbs, 190mg sodium.

INGREDIENTS

- 1 lb chicken breast
- 1 can diced tomatoes
- 1 cup enchilada sauce
- 1 onion, chopped
- 1 can black beans, rinsed
- 1 tsp cumin
- 2 cups low-sodium broth
- 1 cup corn

INSTRUCTIONS

- Place all ingredients in crock pot and cook on low for 7 hours.
- Shred chicken, stir, and top with avocado or low-fat cheese.

13. CROCK POT VENISON & VEGETABLES

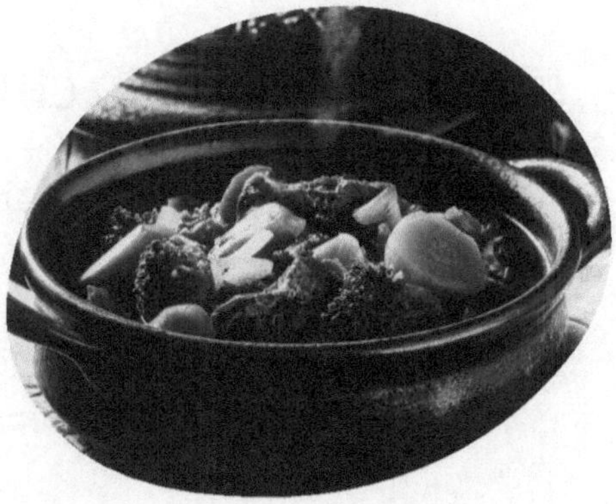

Lean protein and colorful vegetables make this meal hearty

Nutrition: 220 kcal, 27g protein, 5g fat, 10g carbs, 160mg sodium.

INGREDIENTS

- 2 cups venison cubes
- 1 cup carrots
- 1 cup broccoli
- ½ cup onion
- 1 tsp Worcestershire sauce
- ½ tsp soy sauce
- ½ cup water

INSTRUCTIONS

- Add all ingredients to crock pot, stir, and cook on medium for 6 hours.
- Serve with brown rice or steamed potatoes.

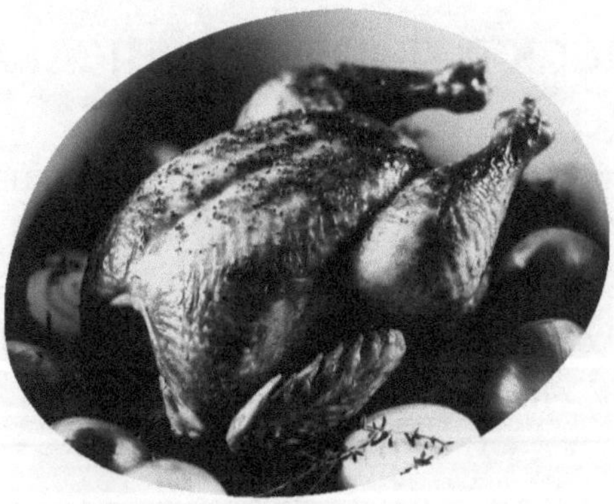

14. ROAST CROCK POT CHICKEN

Simple, flavorful, and perfect for family-style meals.

Nutrition: 240 kcal, 32g protein, 9g fat, 3g carbs, 220mg sodium.

INGREDIENTS

- 1 whole chicken (3–4 lb)
- 1 onion, sliced
- 1 cup low-sodium chicken stock
- 1 tsp paprika
- ½ tsp dried herbs
- 1 garlic clove, minced

INSTRUCTIONS

- Place onion at base of crock pot.
- Add chicken, season with paprika, herbs, and garlic.
- Pour stock over and cook on low for 6 hours until meat pulls away easily.

15. CROCK POT GROUND CHICKEN & BROWN RICE

A complete one-pot meal for effortless nutrition.

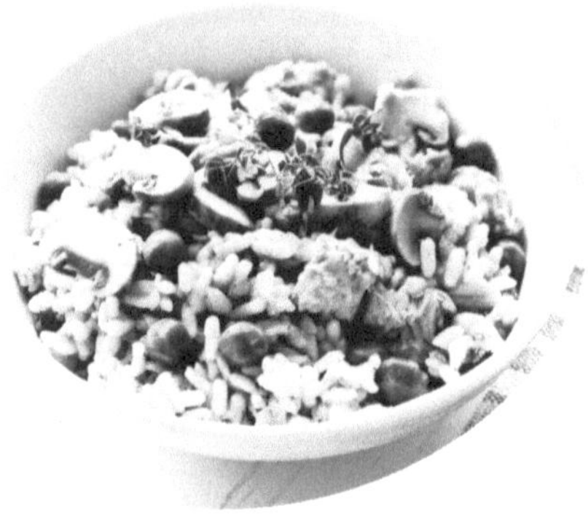

Nutrition: 260 kcal, 22g protein, 6g fat, 31g carbs, 210mg sodium

INGREDIENTS

- 1 lb ground chicken
- 1 cup mushrooms, sliced
- ½ cup celery
- ½ cup onions
- 1 cup peas
- 1 cup low-sodium broth
- 2 cups cooked brown rice

INSTRUCTIONS

- Brown chicken, then place with vegetables and broth in crock pot.
- Cook 3 hours on high.
- Add rice, stir, and heat through before serving.

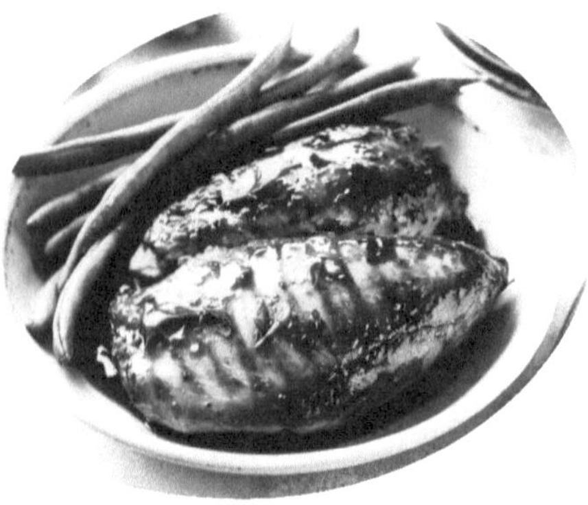

16. CROCK POT PACIFIC CHICKEN

Lightly sweet with a ginger-garlic aroma.

Nutrition: 230 kcal, 28g protein, 5g fat, 11g carbs, 310mg sodium.

INGREDIENTS

- 1 lb chicken breasts
- ½ cup low-sodium soy sauce
- 2 tbsp brown sugar
- 2 tsp grated ginger
- 2 garlic cloves, minced

INSTRUCTIONS

- Combine sauce ingredients in a bowl and pour over chicken in crock pot.
- Cook on low 7 hours until tender.
- Serve with steamed veggies.

17. CROCK POT SEAFOOD STEW

A coastal-style light meal rich in omega-3s.

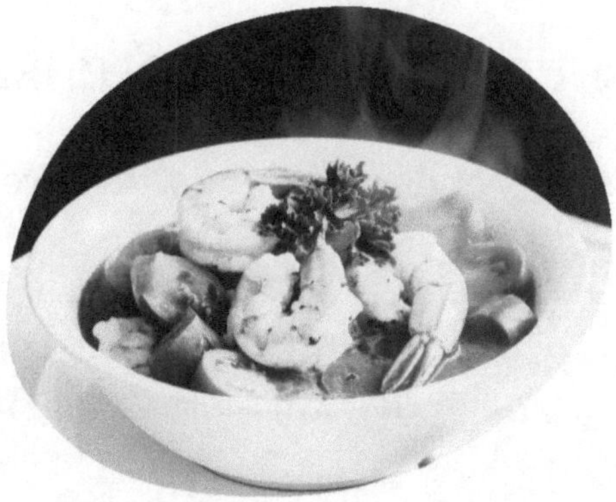

Nutrition: 210 kcal, 25g protein, 7g fat, 10g carbs, 240mg sodium.

INGREDIENTS

- 1 tbsp olive oil
- 1 cup tomatoes, diced
- 1 cup carrots, sliced
- ½ cup bell pepper
- 1 cup low-sodium clam juice
- ½ lb shrimp
- ½ lb cod
- ½ tsp basil

INSTRUCTIONS

- Place all vegetables and juice in crock pot.
- Cook on low 8 hours.
- Add seafood and basil in last 20 minutes until fish flakes easily.
- Serve with parsley garnish.

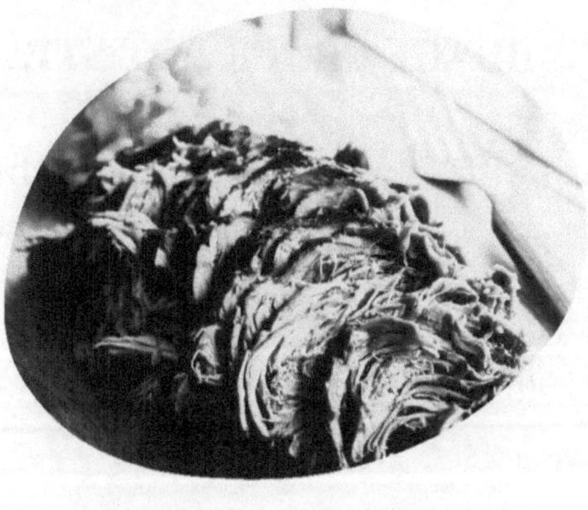

18. BARBEQUE PULLED PORK ROAST

Tender, sweet, and tangy, perfect for gatherings.

Nutrition: 260 kcal, 27g protein, 8g fat, 16g carbs, 220mg sodium.

INGREDIENTS

- 2½ lbs lean pork roast
- 1 cup onion, chopped
- 1 cup tomato sauce
- 2 tbsp vinegar
- 1 tbsp brown sugar
- ½ tsp garlic powder

INSTRUCTIONS

- Combine all ingredients in crock pot, coat pork evenly, and cook on low 7 hours.
- Shred meat and mix with sauce before serving.

19. CROCK POT MAC 'N CHEESE (LIGHT)

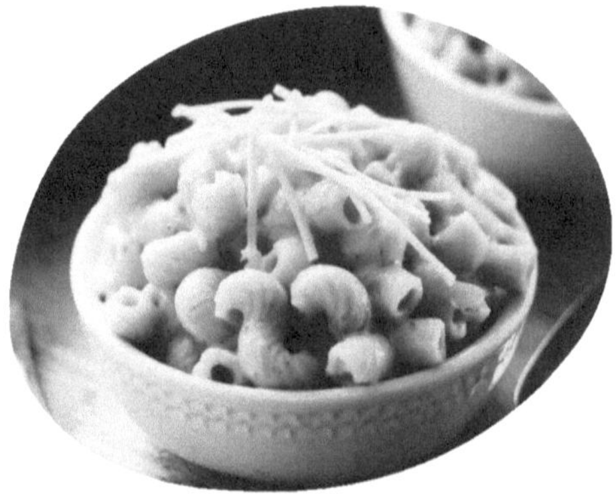

Creamy and comforting with lower sodium and fat.

Nutrition: 230 kcal, 13g protein, 7g fat, 27g carbs, 210mg sodium.

INGREDIENTS

- 8 oz whole wheat pasta
- 1½ cups low-fat milk
- 1 cup low-sodium broth
- 1½ cups reduced-fat cheddar
- ¼ cup chopped onion
- ½ tsp pepper

INSTRUCTIONS

- Add milk, broth, and onion to crock pot.
- Stir in pasta and cheese.
- Cover and cook on low for 3½ hours, stirring halfway.
- Serve warm.

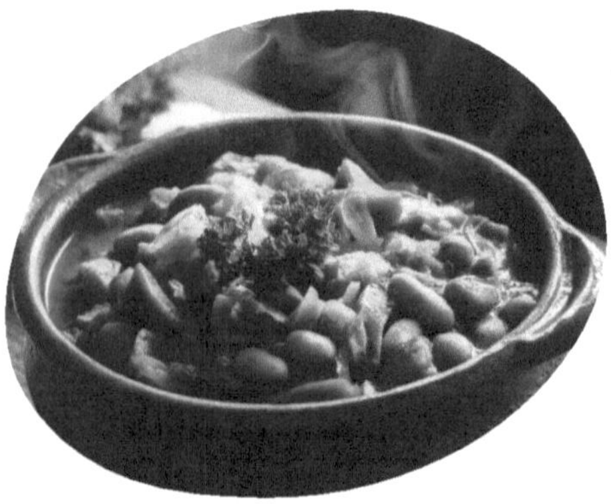

20. IRISH BEAN & CABBAGE CROCK POT STEW

Fiber-rich and anti-inflammatory with a vegetable base.

Nutrition: 190 kcal, 10g protein, 3g fat, 31g carbs, 140mg sodium.

INGREDIENTS

- 1 onion, chopped
- 2 carrots, sliced
- 2 celery stalks, diced
- ½ head cabbage, chopped
- 1 can low-sodium beans
- 4 cups low-sodium broth
- ½ tsp thyme

INSTRUCTIONS

- Combine all ingredients in crock pot and cook on low for 6 hours.
- Stir in beans near end and cook another 30 minutes.
- Serve hot with parsley garnish.

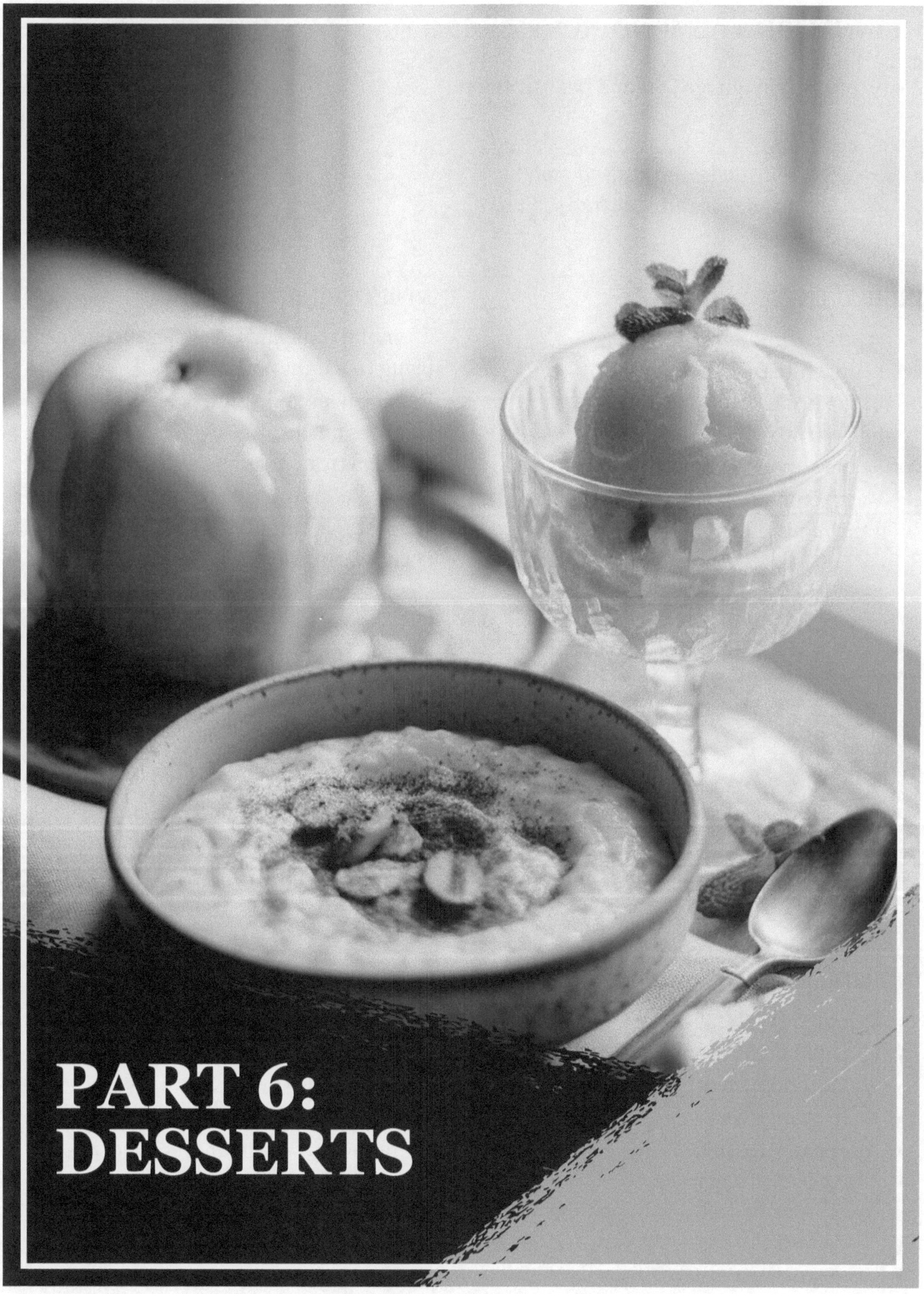

PART 6: DESSERTS

1. CINNAMON & ALMOND RICE PUDDING

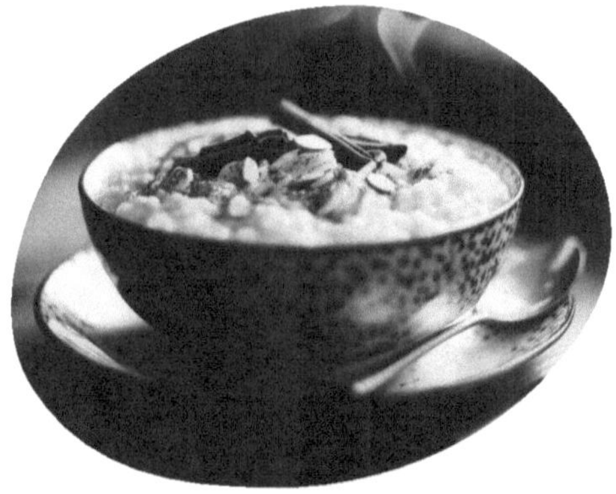

Zesty and rich in omega-3s for a healthy heart.

Nutrition: ~190 kcal; 7g protein; 3g fat; 35g carbs; ~95mg sodium.

INGREDIENTS

- 3 cups 1% milk
- 1 cup white rice
- 3 tbsp honey
- 1 tsp vanilla
- 1/4 tsp almond extract
- 1/4 tsp cinnamon
- 2 tbsp toasted almonds

INSTRUCTIONS

- Combine milk and rice in a saucepan and bring to a light boil.
- Reduce heat and simmer for 25–30 minutes until soft.
- Remove from heat and stir in honey, vanilla, almond extract, and cinnamon.
- Let rest five minutes.
- Serve warm and sprinkle with almonds.

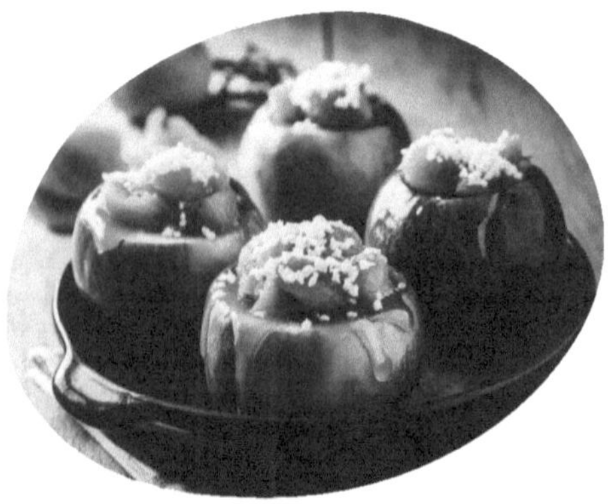

2. STUFFED & BAKED APPLES

Bright, balanced, and full of heart-healthy flavor.

Nutrition: ~170 kcal; 2g protein; 2g fat; 38g carbs; ~40mg sodium.

INGREDIENTS

- 4 Golden Delicious apples
- 1/4 cup flaked coconut
- 1/4 cup chopped dried apricots
- 2 tsp orange zest
- 1/2 cup orange juice
- 1 tbsp brown sugar

INSTRUCTIONS

- Core apples and place in a shallow baking dish.
- Mix coconut, apricots, and zest; stuff evenly into apple centers.
- Combine brown sugar and juice, then pour over apples.
- Cover and bake at 350°F for 25–30 minutes until tender.
- Serve warm or chilled.

3. WATERMELON & LEMON SORBET

Zesty and rich in omega-3s for a healthy heart.

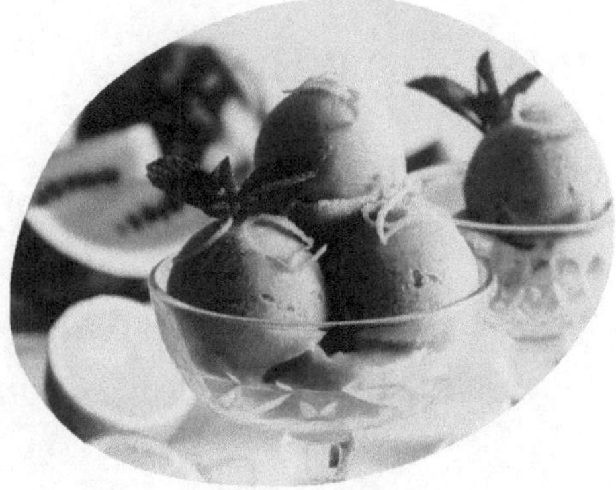

Nutrition: ~85 kcal; 1g protein; 0g fat; 21g carbs; ~10mg sodium.

INGREDIENTS

- 8 cups cubed watermelon
- 2 tbsp fresh lemon juice
- 2 tsp honey

INSTRUCTIONS

- Puree watermelon in a blender until smooth.
- Add lemon juice and honey, stirring gently.
- Freeze in an ice cream maker or container until firm.
- Scoop and serve cold.

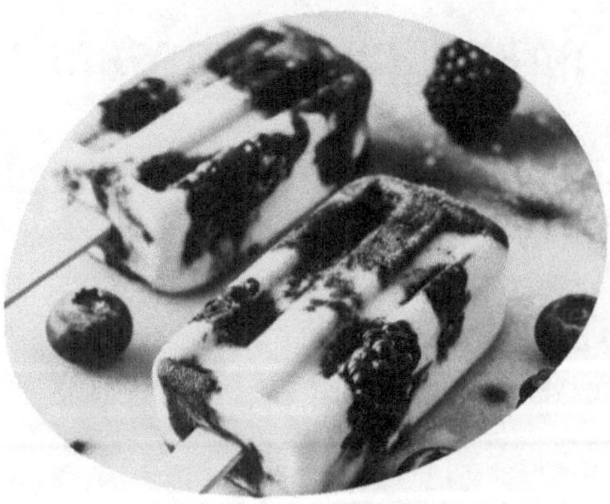

4. BERRY & YOGURT POPSICLES

Fruity frozen delight for sunny afternoons.

Nutrition: ~95 kcal; 5g protein; 1g fat; 17g carbs; ~45mg sodium.

INGREDIENTS

- 1 cup blueberries
- 1 cup blackberries
- 1 cup low-fat plain yogurt
- 1 cup skim milk
- 1 tsp vanilla

INSTRUCTIONS

- Blend berries, yogurt, milk, and vanilla until smooth.
- Pour into molds and freeze for 30 minutes.
- Insert sticks and freeze one hour more until firm.
- Serve cold.

5. PUMPKIN WHIP

Fluffy, spiced, and perfectly light dessert.

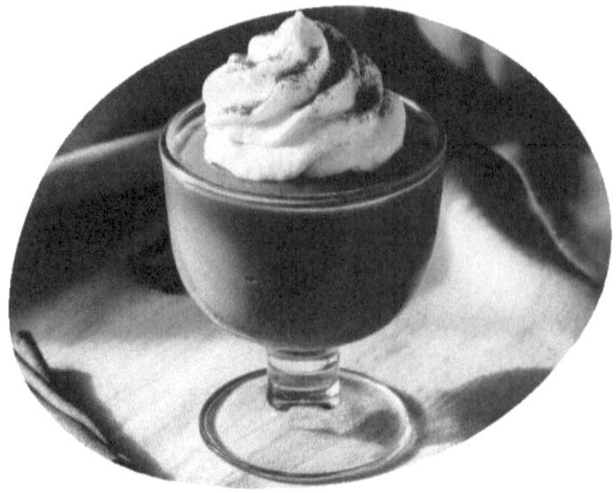

Nutrition: ~120 kcal; 5g protein;
2g fat; 19g carbs; ~140mg sodium.

INGREDIENTS

- 1 package sugar-free cheesecake pudding mix (3.4 oz)
- 1 cup skim milk
- ½ cup solid pumpkin puree
- ½ tsp cinnamon
- ¼ tsp nutmeg
- ½ cup light whipped topping

INSTRUCTIONS

- Whisk milk and pudding until thickened.
- Stir in pumpkin and spices until smooth.
- Fold in whipped topping.
- Chill 30 minutes before serving.

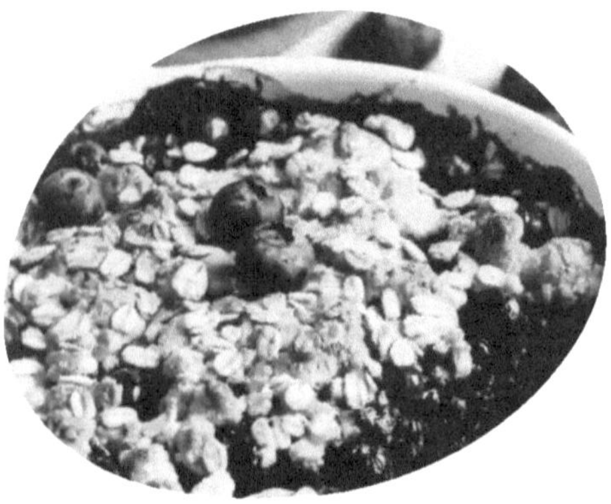

6. BAKED BLUEBERRY BLING

Juicy berries topped with golden crumble.

Nutrition: ~160 kcal; 3g protein;
3g fat; 33g carbs; ~35mg sodium.

INGREDIENTS

- 3 cups blueberries
- 2 tsp butter
- 1 tbsp flour
- 1 tbsp brown sugar
- ½ cup oats
- ½ tsp cinnamon

INSTRUCTIONS

- Preheat oven to 375°F.
- Combine flour, oats, sugar, and cinnamon in a bowl.
- Add softened butter and mix until crumbly.
- Spread blueberries in dish and sprinkle topping.
- Bake 20 minutes and serve warm.

7. PINA COLADA POPSICLES

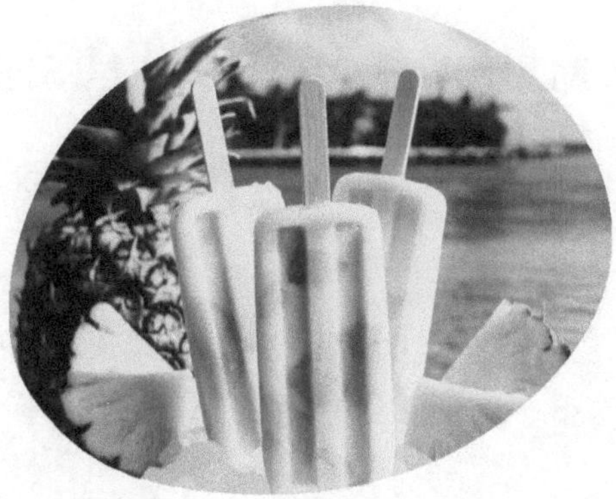

Tropical flavor that cools and refreshes.

Nutrition: ~90 kcal; 1g protein; 2g fat; 17g carbs; ~25mg sodium.

INGREDIENTS

- 1 cup diced pineapple
- 1/4 cup pineapple juice
- 1/2 cup light coconut milk
- 1 tsp coconut extract
- 1 tsp honey

INSTRUCTIONS

- Blend all ingredients until smooth.
- Pour into molds and freeze for 2 hours.
- Serve chilled.

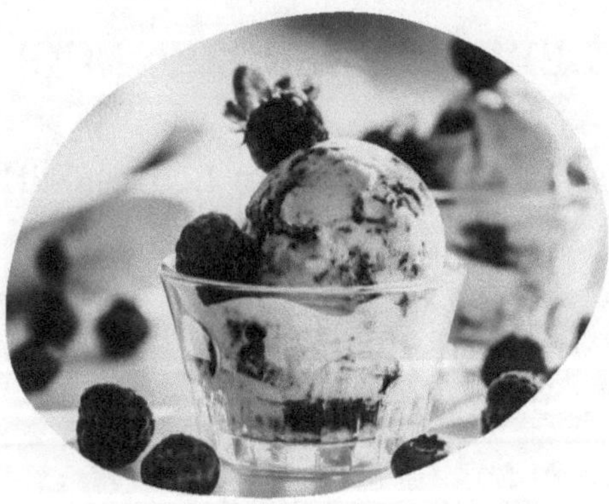

8. BERRY-BANANA GUILT-FREE ICE CREAM

Smooth, fruity, and naturally dairy-free treat.

Nutrition: ~130 kcal; 3g protein; 1g fat; 29g carbs; ~40mg sodium.

INGREDIENTS

- 3 large frozen bananas
- 1 cup frozen berries
- 1/2 cup skim milk
- 1 tsp vanilla

INSTRUCTIONS

- Add bananas, milk, and vanilla to blender.
- Process until creamy.
- Add berries and pulse lightly for texture.
- Serve immediately or freeze for later.

9. MELON & ORANGE SLUSHY

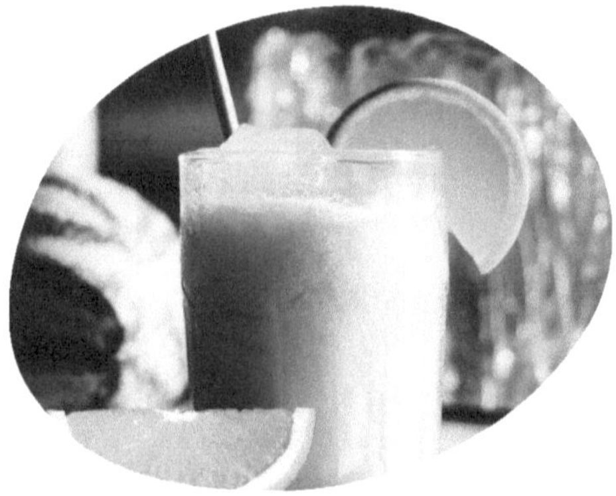

Quick, chilled blend of fruit and zest.

Nutrition: ~75 kcal; 1g protein; 0g fat; 18g carbs; ~20mg sodium.

INGREDIENTS

- 5 ice cubes
- 4 cups cubed ripe cantaloupe
- 1/4 cup orange juice
- 1 tsp honey

INSTRUCTIONS

- Add all ingredients to blender.
- Blend for 10 seconds until smooth and slushy.
- Serve immediately while cold.

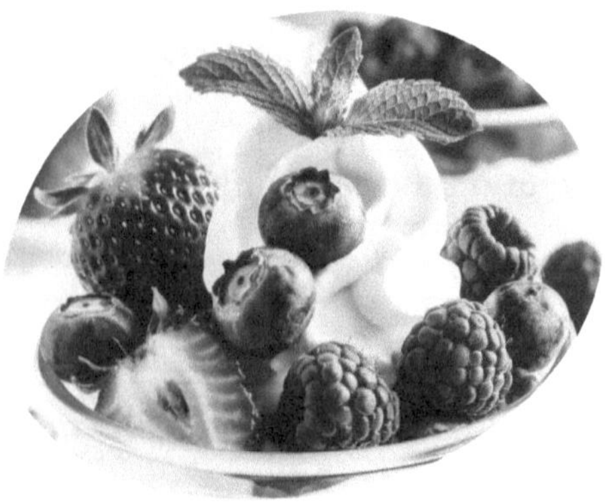

10. SUMMER BERRIES IN FROZEN YOGURT

Bright, antioxidant-rich dessert for heart health.

Nutrition: ~155 kcal; 6g protein; 2g fat; 29g carbs; ~70mg sodium.

INGREDIENTS

- 1 cup sliced strawberries
- 1 cup blueberries
- 1 cup raspberries
- 1 tsp orange zest
- 3 tbsp orange juice
- 2 cups low-fat vanilla frozen yogurt

INSTRUCTIONS

- Mix berries with juice and zest.
- Chill for 2 hours.
- Scoop frozen yogurt into bowls.
- Top with the berry mixture.

11. CRANBERRY-WATERMELON AGUA FRESCA

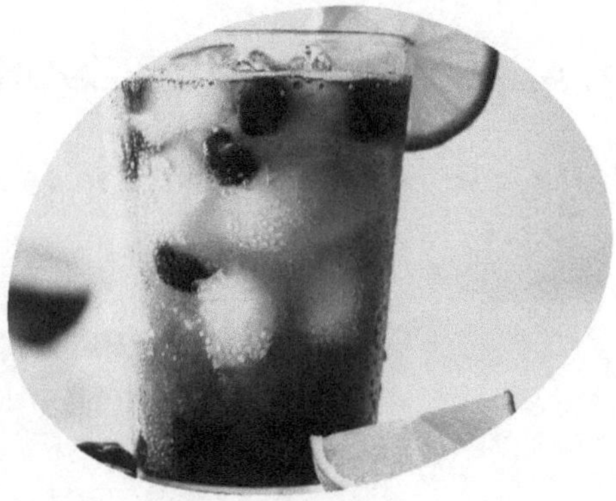

Light, fruity drink with a tangy finish.

Nutrition: ~65 kcal; 1g protein; 0g fat; 16g carbs; ~25mg sodium.

INGREDIENTS

- 7 cups cubed watermelon
- 1 cup cranberry juice
- 1/4 cup lime juice

INSTRUCTIONS

- Blend watermelon until smooth and strain.
- Combine with cranberry and lime juice.
- Refrigerate for 1 hour.
- Serve over ice.

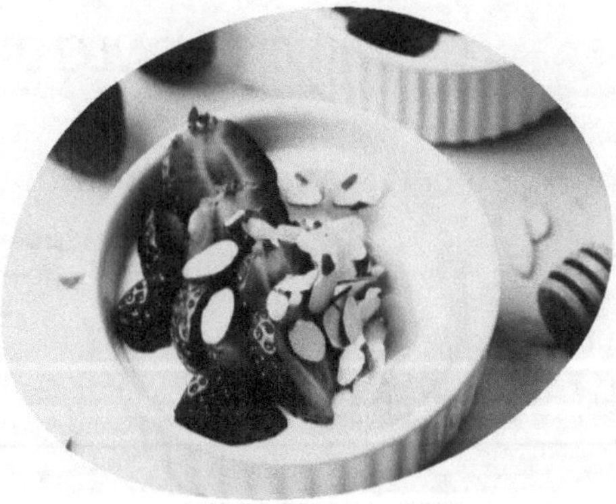

12. FRESH STRAWBERRIES & HONEY YOGURT

Simple, protein-rich fruit and yogurt pairing.

Nutrition: ~120 kcal; 8g protein; 3g fat; 16g carbs; ~55mg sodium.

INGREDIENTS

- 1 pint fresh strawberries, sliced
- 3 cups plain low-fat yogurt
- 4 tsp honey
- 2 tbsp toasted almonds

INSTRUCTIONS

- Place yogurt in serving bowls.
- Top with strawberries.
- Drizzle honey and sprinkle almonds.
- Serve chilled.

13. ALMOND & TAHINI COOKIES

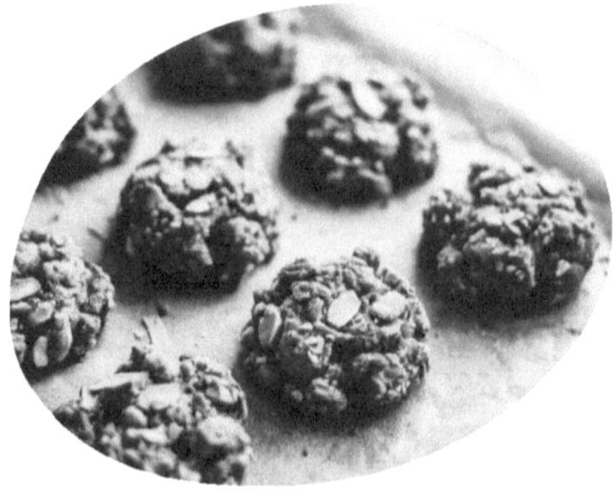

Nutty, soft cookies with a wholesome twist.

Nutrition: ~95 kcal; 2g protein; 5g fat; 10g carbs; ~45mg sodium.

INGREDIENTS

- 1 cup whole wheat flour
- ½ cup almond meal
- 3 tbsp butter
- ¼ cup sugar
- 2 tbsp tahini
- ½ tsp vanilla extract
- 2 tbsp water

INSTRUCTIONS

- Preheat oven to 350°F.
- Mix all ingredients into a soft dough.
- Form small balls, flatten slightly.
- Bake 12 minutes until golden.
- Cool and serve.

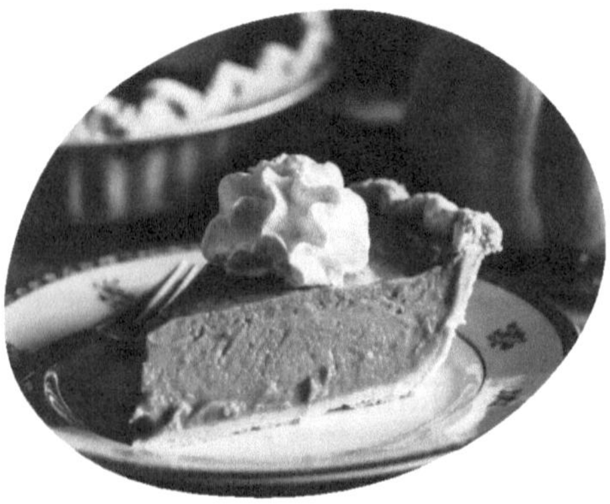

14. SWEET POTATO PIE

Smooth, spiced pie for cozy evenings.

Nutrition: ~190 kcal; 5g protein; 6g fat; 30g carbs; ~140mg sodium.

INGREDIENTS

- 1 cup mashed sweet potato
- ½ cup brown sugar
- ¼ tsp cinnamon
- Pinch nutmeg
- 2 eggs
- ¼ cup milk
- 1 tsp melted butter
- 1 prepared pie crust

INSTRUCTIONS

- Preheat oven to 400°F.
- Combine potato, sugar, and spices.
- Whisk eggs, milk, and butter separately.
- Blend both mixtures.
- Pour into crust and bake 40–45 minutes until set.

15. APPLE CRUMBLE PIE

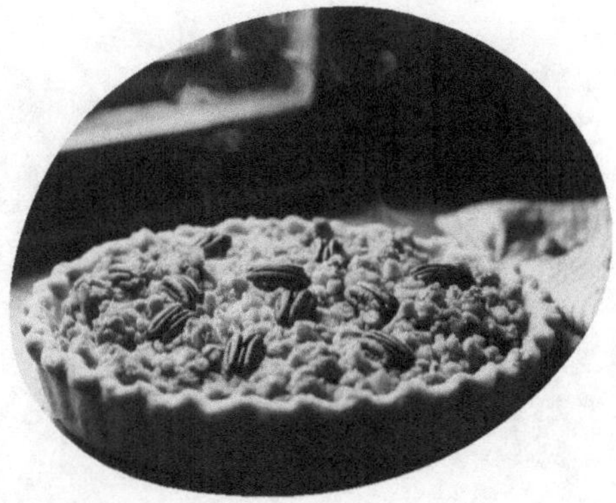

Classic comfort with heart-smart ingredients.

Nutrition: ~210 kcal; 3g protein; 7g fat; 36g carbs; ~75mg sodium.

INGREDIENTS

- 3 apples, peeled and chopped
- 1/2 cup oats
- 1/4 cup brown sugar
- 1/4 cup flour
- 1/4 cup chopped pecans
- 1/2 tsp cinnamon
- 2 tbsp light butter

INSTRUCTIONS

- Preheat oven to 375°F.
- Place apples in a pie dish.
- Mix oats, sugar, flour, pecans, and cinnamon.
- Cut in butter until crumbly.
- Sprinkle over apples and bake 35–40 minutes.

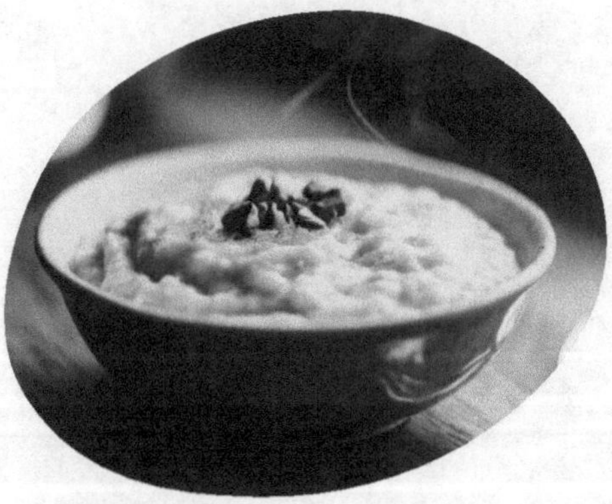

16. ORANGE RICE PUDDING

Creamy citrus rice pudding with subtle zest.

Nutrition: ~180 kcal; 7g protein; 3g fat; 32g carbs; ~90mg sodium.

INGREDIENTS

- 3/4 cup basmati rice
- 2 large oranges
- 4 cups fat-free evaporated milk
- 1/4 cup low-fat condensed milk
- 3 tbsp sugar
- 1/2 tsp orange zest
- 2 tbsp chopped pistachios (optional)

INSTRUCTIONS

- Cook rice in 2 cups of water until tender.
- Grate zest from one orange and squeeze juice; set aside.
- Combine cooked rice with milk, condensed milk, zest, juice, and sugar.
- Simmer over medium heat, stirring often, until creamy.
- Serve warm or chilled, topped with pistachios.

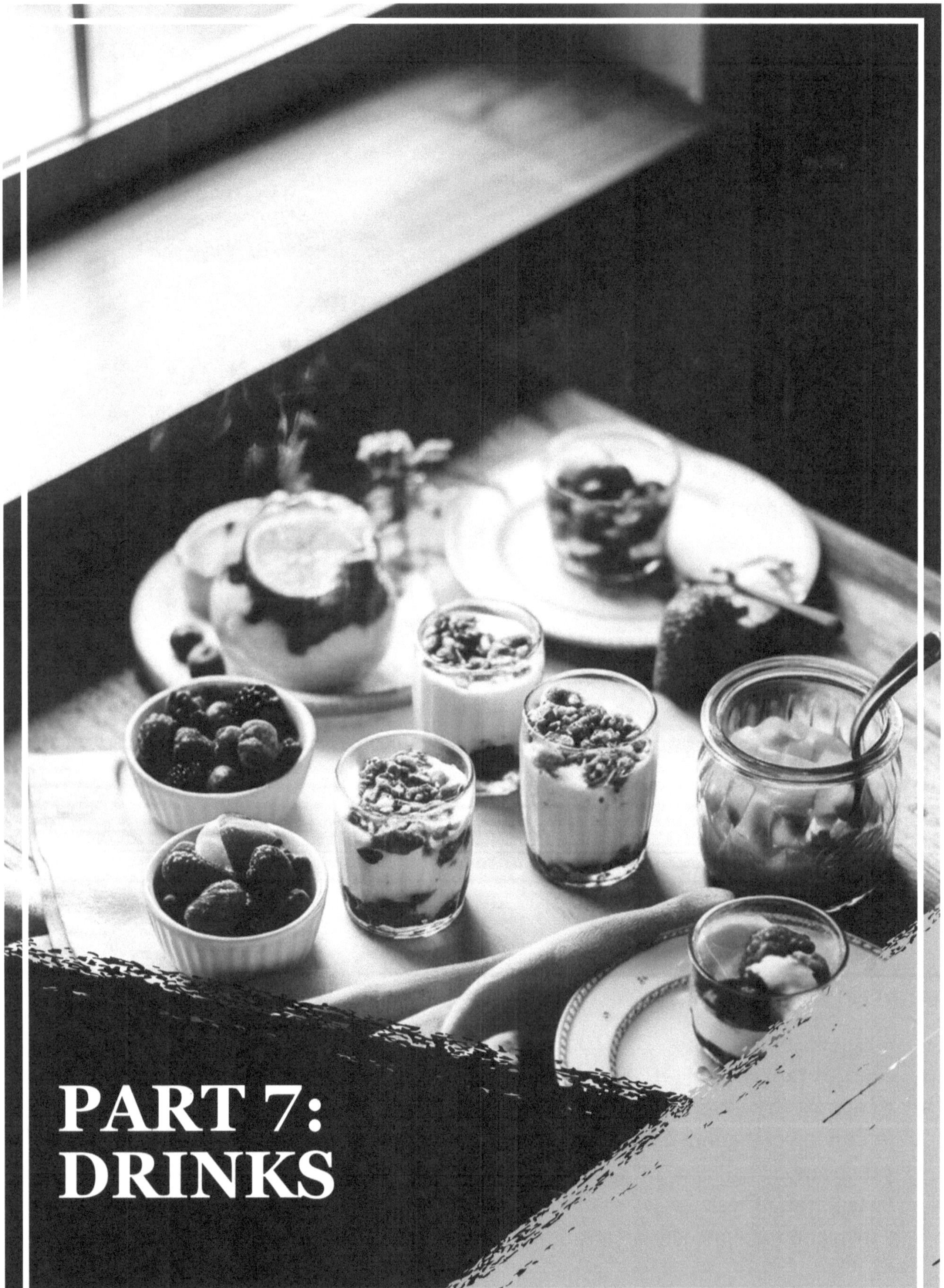

PART 7: DRINKS

1. BERRY MIX SMOOTHIE

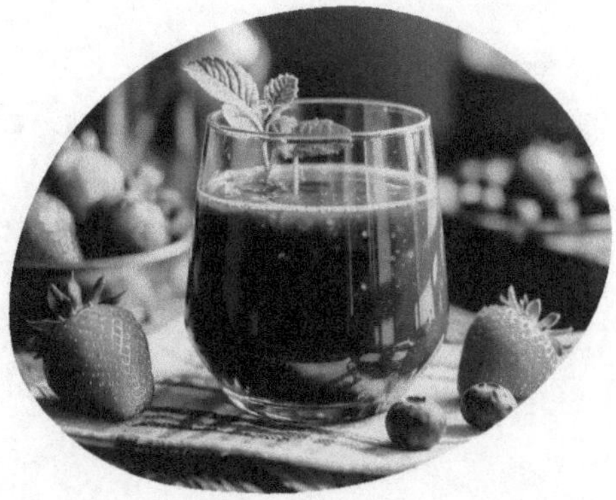

Refreshing and rich in antioxidants.

Nutrition: ~110 kcal; 3g protein; 2g fat; 20g carbs; ~35mg sodium.

INGREDIENTS

- 1½ cups strawberries
- ½ cup blueberries
- ⅓ cup water or vanilla yogurt
- ¼ tsp vanilla extract
- 1 tbsp flaxseed

INSTRUCTIONS

- Place all ingredients in a blender.
- Process until smooth in consistency.
- Serve garnished with strawberries if desired.

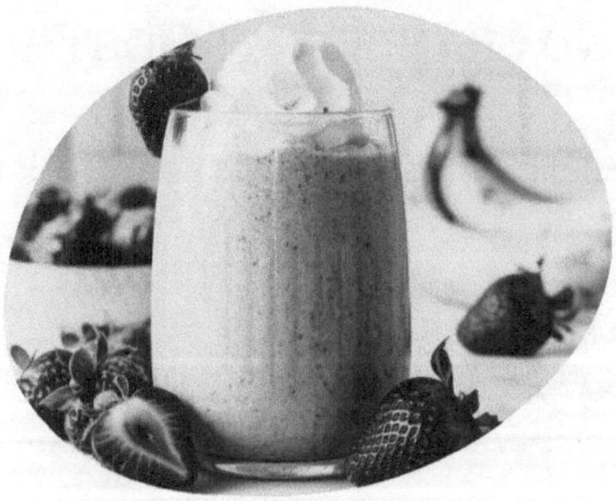

2. SOY FRUIT SMOOTHIE

Creamy, sweet, and protein-packed.

Nutrition: ~150 kcal; 6g protein; 3g fat; 26g carbs; ~60mg sodium.

INGREDIENTS

- 2 cups strawberries, halved
- 1½ cups vanilla low-fat soy milk
- 1½ tbsp honey
- ½ tsp vanilla extract
- 1 banana, sliced
- 1 cup fat-free whipped topping

INSTRUCTIONS

- Place strawberries, milk, honey, vanilla, and banana in a blender.
- Blend until smooth.
- Top each glass with whipped topping.

3. CANTALOUPE AND ORANGE SMOOTHIE

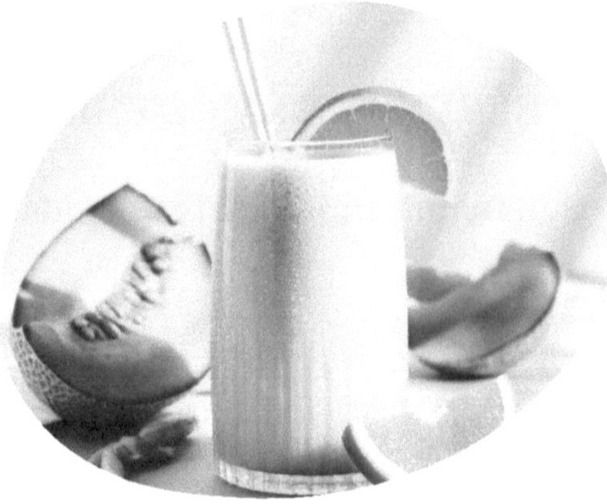

A light citrus blend for summer days.

Nutrition: ~95 kcal; 2g protein; 0g fat; 22g carbs; ~30mg sodium.

INGREDIENTS

- 1 small orange, peeled and sectioned
- 1/4 cantaloupe, chopped
- 1/2 frozen banana
- 6 ice cubes

INSTRUCTIONS

- Add all ingredients to a blender.
- Blend until smooth and creamy.
- Serve immediately.

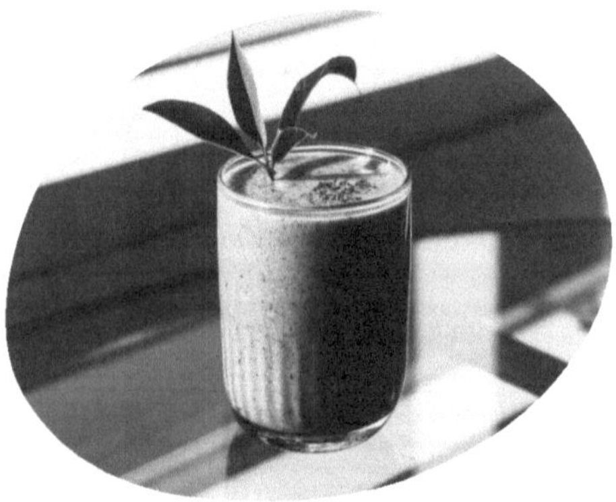

4. GREEN TEA AND CRANBERRY SMOOTHIE

Energizing blend with a tart finish.

Nutrition: ~130 kcal; 2g protein; 1g fat; 29g carbs; ~40mg sodium.

INGREDIENTS

- 1/2 cup frozen cranberries
- 1/4 cup frozen blueberries
- 1/2 cup frozen blackberries
- 1 banana
- 1/2 cup brewed green tea, cooled
- 1/4 cup plain soy milk
- 2 tbsp honey

INSTRUCTIONS

- Combine all ingredients in a blender.
- Blend until smooth in consistency.
- Pour into chilled glasses.

5. ORANGE STRAWBERRY TWIRL

A tangy, creamy twist on fruit flavor.

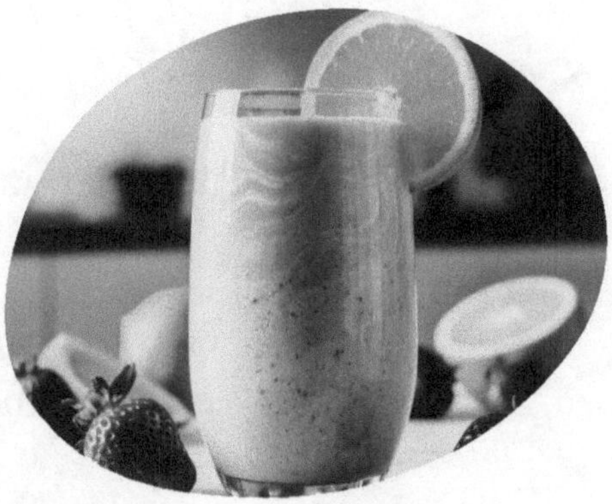

Nutrition: ~160 kcal; 6g protein; 1g fat; 30g carbs; ~55mg sodium.

INGREDIENTS

- 2 packages frozen strawberries in light syrup (10 oz each)
- 1 container plain low-fat yogurt (6 oz)
- 1 cup fresh orange juice
- 1 cup fat-free milk

INSTRUCTIONS

- Add all ingredients to blender.
- Blend until smooth and pour into glasses.
- Serve chilled.

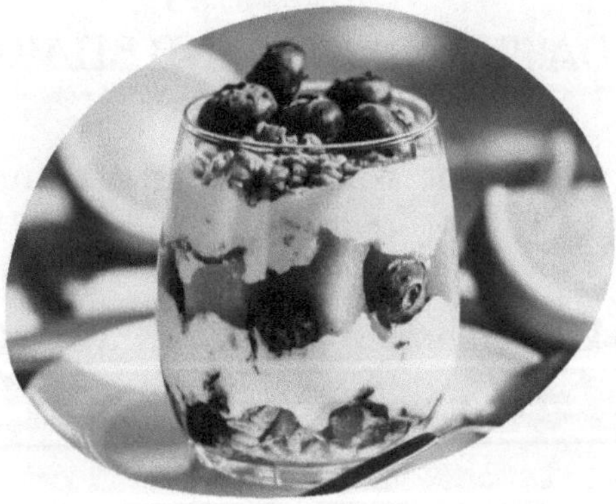

6. BERRY ORANGE MIX

Sweet layers of fruit and creamy yogurt.

Nutrition: ~190 kcal; 8g protein; 4g fat; 32g carbs; ~75mg sodium.

INGREDIENTS

- 3 medium oranges, peeled
- 1 container 2% Greek yogurt (7 oz)
- 2 tbsp honey
- ½ tsp orange zest
- ½ tsp vanilla extract
- 1 cup blueberries
- 1 cup granola

INSTRUCTIONS

- Mix yogurt, honey, zest, and vanilla.
- Layer oranges, yogurt, blueberries, and granola in glasses.
- Repeat layers and serve.

7. SMOOTHIE SUNRAY

Bright and fruity morning energizer.

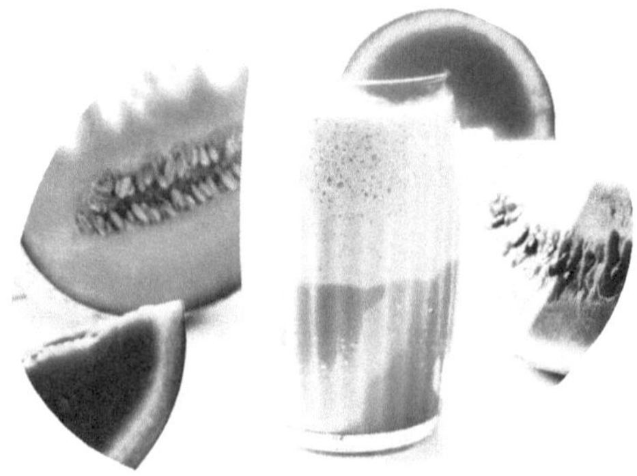

Nutrition: ~120 kcal; 4g protein; 1g fat; 25g carbs; ~40mg sodium.

INGREDIENTS

- 1½ cups diced watermelon
- 1 cup diced cantaloupe
- ½ cup low-fat yogurt
- ¼ cup orange juice

INSTRUCTIONS

- Blend watermelon until smooth and pour into glasses.
- Blend cantaloupe, yogurt, and juice separately.
- Pour over watermelon layer and serve.

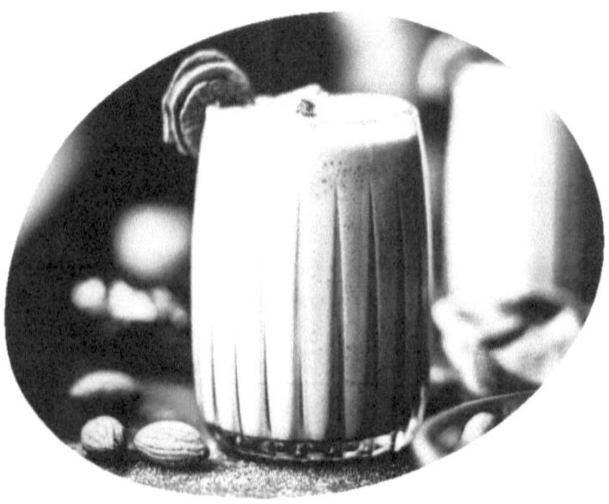

8. DATE AND ALMOND SHAKE

Naturally sweet, fiber-rich nutty drink.

Nutrition: ~180 kcal; 7g protein; 4g fat; 32g carbs; ~65mg sodium.

INGREDIENTS

- ⅓ cup chopped dates
- 2 tbsp warm water
- 2 cups vanilla almond milk
- ½ cup fat-free vanilla yogurt
- 1 frozen banana
- ⅛ tsp nutmeg
- 4 ice cubes

INSTRUCTIONS

- Soak dates in warm water for 10 minutes.
- Blend soaked dates, milk, yogurt, banana, nutmeg, and ice.
- Blend until smooth and sprinkle nutmeg on top.

9. MANGO AND AVOCADO SMOOTHIE SURPRISE

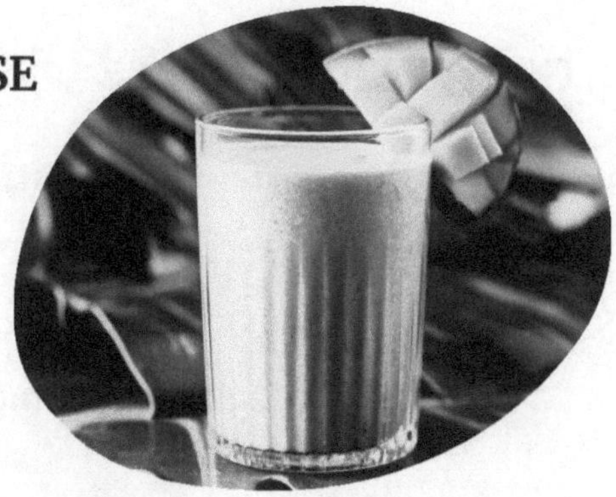

Creamy tropical blend for balanced energy.

Nutrition: ~140 kcal; 4g protein; 5g fat; 20g carbs; ~50mg sodium.

INGREDIENTS

- 1/4 cup mango cubes
- 1/4 cup mashed avocado
- 1/2 cup mango juice
- 1/4 cup fat-free vanilla yogurt
- 1 tbsp lime juice
- 1 tbsp honey
- 6 ice cubes

INSTRUCTIONS

- Combine all ingredients in a blender.
- Blend until smooth and creamy.
- Pour into glasses and garnish with mango.

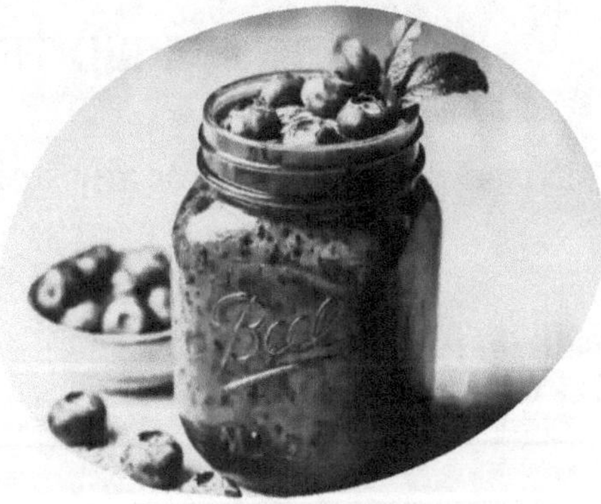

10. NOT TOO SWEET BLUEBERRY SMOOTHIE

Mildly sweet and omega-rich breakfast drink.

Nutrition: ~120 kcal; 5g protein; 4g fat; 16g carbs; ~55mg sodium.

INGREDIENTS

- 1 cup frozen unsweetened blueberries
- 1 tbsp flaxseed oil
- 1 cup skim milk

INSTRUCTIONS

- Place blueberries in blender.
- Add milk and blend until smooth.
- Stir in flaxseed oil and serve immediately.

11. GOLDEN ICED LATTE

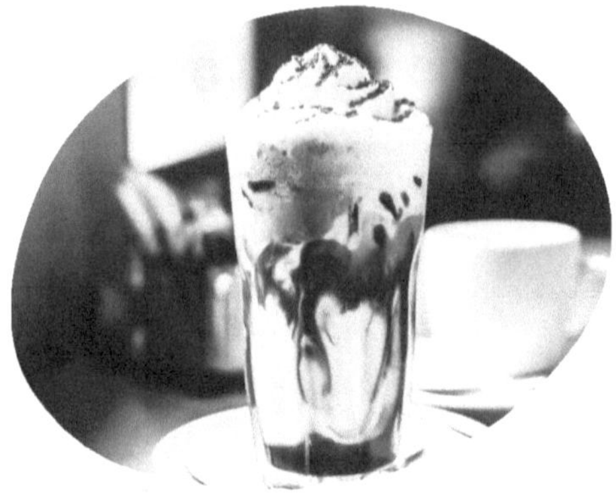

Smooth, mellow coffee with a nutty note.

Nutrition: ~95 kcal; 6g protein; 2g fat; 12g carbs; ~70mg sodium.

INGREDIENTS

- 2 cups decaf espresso, cooled
- 2 tbsp brown sugar
- 1½ cups fat-free milk
- 2 tbsp sugar-free almond syrup
- Ice cubes
- 1 cup fat-free whipped topping
- 1 tsp ground espresso beans

INSTRUCTIONS

- Mix coffee, sugar, milk, and almond syrup in a pitcher.
- Chill for 30 minutes.
- Pour over ice, top with whipped cream, and sprinkle espresso powder.

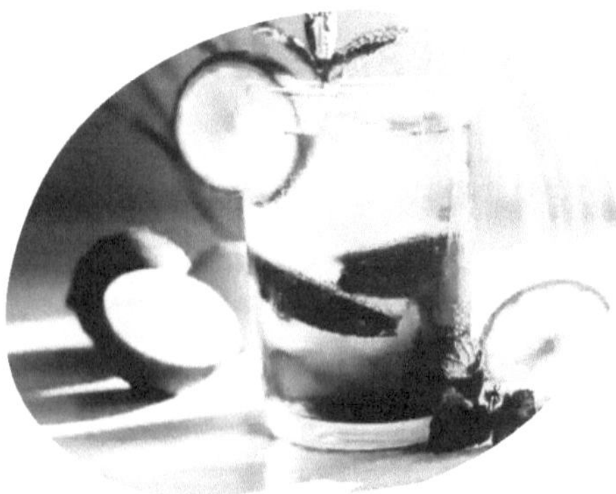

12. MINTY ICED TEA

Cooling, mint-infused refreshment for any time.

Nutrition: ~35 kcal; 0g protein; 0g fat; 8g carbs; ~10mg sodium.

INGREDIENTS

- 1 cup brewed unsweetened tea, cooled
- 2 tbsp lime juice
- 2 tbsp fresh mint leaves
- 5 ice cubes
- Sugar substitute, to taste

INSTRUCTIONS

- Blend mint, lime juice, and ice cubes.
- Add tea and process until smooth.
- Mix in sweetener as desired and serve chilled.

13. BREAKFAST MOJITO

Citrus-mint drink that boosts morning freshness.

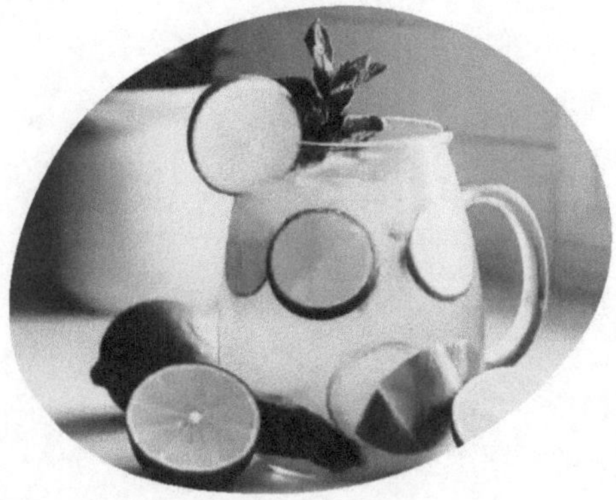

Nutrition: ~130 kcal; 1g protein; 0g fat; 32g carbs; ~25mg sodium.

INGREDIENTS

- 1/2 cup dark honey
- 1/2 cup fresh lime juice
- 1/2 cup fresh mint leaves
- 2 cups grapefruit juice
- 2 cups orange juice
- 2 tsp lime zest
- 1 lime, sliced

INSTRUCTIONS

- Boil honey and lime juice.
- Add mint leaves and steep for 5 minutes.
- Strain and cool.
- Mix syrup with juices and zest.
- Serve over ice with lime slice.

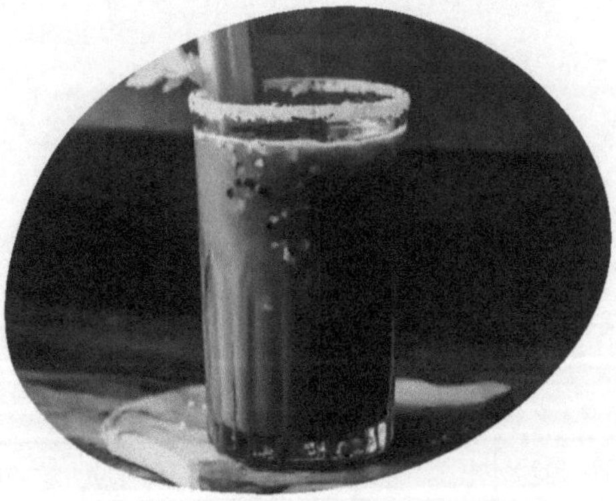

14. SPICY TOMATO SIPPER

Savory, low-sodium drink with a tangy bite.

Nutrition: ~70 kcal; 2g protein; 0g fat; 13g carbs; ~120mg sodium.

INGREDIENTS

- 2 cups low-sodium tomato juice
- 2 tbsp lime juice
- 1 tsp Worcestershire sauce
- 1/2 tsp horseradish
- Few drops hot sauce
- Ice cubes
- Celery sticks (optional)

INSTRUCTIONS

- Combine all ingredients and stir well.
- Pour over ice cubes in tall glasses.
- Garnish with celery stick if desired.

DAILY MEAL PLANNER

BREAKFAST

- [ ]
- [ ]
- [ ]

LUNCH

- [ ]
- [ ]
- [ ]

DINNER

- [ ]
- [ ]
- [ ]

DASH DIET GROCERY LIST

VEGETABLES

Fresh or frozen vegetables such as spinach, broccoli, carrots, kale, zucchini, sweet potatoes, and peppers. Aim for four to five servings daily to support circulation and reduce inflammation.

FRUITS

Apples, bananas, oranges, berries, and melons provide potassium and fiber that assist in maintaining healthy blood pressure.

WHOLE

Brown rice, oats, quinoa, barley, and whole-grain pasta or bread help keep you full and balance blood sugar levels.

LEAN PROTEINS

Skinless poultry, fish, and small portions of lean beef or pork offer essential amino acids without excess fat.

LOW-FAT OR NO-FAT DAIRY

Yogurt, milk, and cheese alternatives strengthen bones while keeping saturated fat low.

NUTS AND SEEDS

Almonds, walnuts, sunflower seeds, and chia seeds are packed with healthy fats, magnesium, and plant protein.

LEGUMES

Beans, peas, and lentils are great vegetarian sources of protein and fiber, perfect for soft food diets or easy-to-chew meals.

HEALTHY OILS

Olive oil and avocado oil provide heart smart fats that reduce cholesterol and boost vitality.